Praise for D

"Defying Mental Illness provides what's needed most: a lucid and more than adequate introduction to mental illness."

— NAMI *E-Advocate*

A Top 20 Book for Parents and Teachers of Children with Special Needs

"It is easy to understand and complete so it is suitable for people in recovery, caregivers, faith-based, church and community outreach workers who work in mental health. Readers will appreciate the chapters on finding treatment, paying for mental health care, housing, employment and disability, involuntary hospitalization, the criminal justice system, and links to allies and advocacy groups.

"The case studies describing a few journeys towards recovery bring hope to the readers."

— Lorna D'Entremont, *Special Needs Book Review*

"This book could be called "Demystifying Mental Illness." The authors have taken the mystery out of mental illness along with the technical jargon . . . *Defying Mental Illness* pulls multiple areas of information together into one easy read. I am a special education teacher and will use this as a go-to reference for the future."

— Five-star review on Amazon

"I think this book is an excellent companion. It is well-researched, well-written, and clear. My congratulations and thanks to the authors for providing an accessible manual that I can recommend as a concrete resource to anyone needing clear guidelines about mental illness, its effect on the family, and the recovery process.

"They state, in the introduction, that the goal was to write "a book that is not too technical, and suitable for community outreach work." This is beautifully accomplished."

—Randye Kaye, author of *Ben Behind His Voices*

"As a practicing psychologist I am very impressed with *Defying Mental Illness*. We have too few books on the market that really take the sting out of what can be a frightening situation . . . I like the fact that the book is such an easy read and yet so complete. Every resource facility out there, including police stations, schools, doctor's offices, community centers, etc. should have this book in their library or easily accessible in a waiting room, a shelf in an interviewer's office, etc."

– Dr. Barbara Becker Holstein

"*Defying Mental Illness* encourages doing what one can to answer illness and help those who struggle find the strength to live their lives. . . . a useful reference and much recommended reading for health and spirituality collections."

– *Midwest Book Review*

RECOVERY STARTS WITH FOUR QUESTIONS.

What helps you make the most of your talents?

How can you reduce the areas where you are vulnerable?

How can you improve your ability to cope with stress?

How can you deal with the risk of something going wrong?

Focused on strengths, *Defying Mental Illness* helps people with mental illness and family members work together as allies.

The book covers mental health disorders, childhood behavioral health, substance abuse, medication, disability programs, violence, hospitalization, guardianship, suicide prevention – and more.

Revised and updated for 2014.

DEFYING MENTAL ILLNESS

Finding Recovery with Community Resources and Family Support

2014 Edition

Paul Komarek
and Andrea Schroer

CHURCH BASEMENT PRESS

Defying Mental Illness: Finding Recovery with Community Resources and Family Support 2014 Edition

By Paul Komarek and Andrea Schroer

Published by
Church Basement Press
4335 Pitts Ave.
Cincinnati, OH 45223
(513) 541-1550
www.churchbasement.net

A Note on Sources

Material from *You Are Not Alone: NAMI Ohio Family and Consumer Resource Guide* is used by permission of NAMI Ohio. If we have failed to identify a source, please contact us so we can credit the author properly in future editions of this publication.

Important Disclaimer

This book is intended for general educational purposes only. It does not substitute for individual medical advice from your doctor or legal advice from your lawyer. Please consult your doctor or lawyer for advice on your individual situation.

DEFYING MENTAL ILLNESS

In a world where there is so much to be done, I felt strongly impressed that there must be something for me to do.

– Dorothea Dix

TABLE OF CONTENTS

CHILD AND ADOLESCENT MENTAL HEALTH 115

PROGRESSING THROUGH ADULTHOOD... 137

PART TWO ALLIES FOR RECOVERY 147

FINDING ALLIES 149

FIGHTING FOR FAMILIES 151

ABOUT THE 2014 EDITION

Human development and social learning have emerged as key themes in this edition of *Defying Mental Illness.*

Also in this edition

- Additional emphasis on trauma and its effects

- Revised chapters on suicide prevention, violence, and crisis response

- The Safe Zone System, a method for balancing safety with a person's need to extend their range and build capacity.

- New material on informed consent and person-centered strength-based care

- New material relating to disability through the lifespan

- New material on addiction, addiction treatment, and addiction recovery programs

- Nonclinical resources for addressing destructive thought patterns, and for discovering a person's key strengths

- Brief comments about the transition currently underway in the U.S. healthcare system

Please contact the author if you have suggestions about what to include in a future update.

The *Defying Mental Illness* website at **www.DefyingMentalIllness.net** includes helpful videos, downloadable worksheets, and links to additional resources.

INTRODUCTION

Mental illness means a struggle, whether it is one's own illness, a friend's illness or a family member's illness. Still, there is a real basis for hope. People with mental illness can and do recover from these disorders. Symptoms can be reduced or completely eliminated. Even when symptoms persist, people can rebuild their capacity to live meaningfully, to work, and to help others.

No one should minimize the challenges of mental illness. Like many other severe and chronic disorders, mental illness devastates people with symptoms, and blasts family, friends and co-workers too. Mental illness causes puzzling episodes of troublesome behavior. Financial problems, career disruption, conflict at school, and involvement with the criminal justice system may follow. Nevertheless, surrendering to mental illness can be tragic, even fatal.

This book relies on insights gained through the authors' own experience, and from a variety of sources we trust. We are teachers, not medical people. We have worked in social service agencies. We have seen the need for a book that is not too technical, yet suitable for a quick reference or for community outreach work.

The authors know many people who have made it through the struggle with mental illness, and many family members and professionals who have supported people with difficult conditions. They have come to terms with mental illness, faced every kind of disorder, and dealt with every kind of treatment. They have rebuilt lives, repaired family relationships, and achieved meaningful success.

You can accomplish this too.

DEFYING MENTAL ILLNESS

Mental illness brings such chaos. People lose energy, or lose connection with reality, or self-destruct. Family life is shattered. When mental illness hits the news, the news is mostly tragic.

Reckoning with mental illness, facing up to the challenge, requires powerful strategies. The author John Carmody has identified what he calls the universal human toolkit for handling trouble. Carmody suggests five techniques: thinking, feeling, sharing, determination, and prayer. Many people who have experienced mental illness or who have cared for a friend or relative have used these tools to find consolation and a way to move forward.

Defying Mental Illness focuses more on the nuts and bolts. It aims to make mental illness topics approachable, and to help readers recognize patterns and make good decisions no matter how mental illness affects their lives. People retain many capacities even when they are experiencing difficult symptoms, so *Defying Mental Illness* is a positive strategy, one that build on strengths.

Mental illness is a biopsychosocial phenomenon, with biological, psychological, and social components. This book covers all three components, especially the social aspects. Nonclinicians – family, friends, neighbors, and communities – directly affect mental health. Improving daily life is a key to mental illness prevention. Ordinary support keeps people motivated and committed as they work through health challenges. And everyone has a role in keeping people safe in the face of elevated risk.

The book introduces enough medical vocabulary and background information to help people understand what is happening and make appropriate decisions about treatment, yet it mostly relies on non-clinical concepts like thinking, feeling, safety, and risk. In areas where there is conflict, the book attempts to activate everyone's best judgment, and highlights options that keep people working together in difficult circumstances.

Even though this book covers some very challenging topics such as suicide, trauma, and violence, at its heart *Defying Mental Illness* is about how to recover and how to help people live safe, meaningful, successful lives, not how to have a disease.

THE *DEFYING MENTAL ILLNESS* STRATEGY

Defying Mental Illness combines learning, relationships, resources, planning, and action –elements drawn from the innate human toolkit – into a five-step strategy

1. Learn about what you are facing. You will need basic information about what is happening, and what can help. Try to understand what others are experiencing. Expect to encounter conflict and uncertainty as you gather information. The subject matter can become extremely complex. Find your path by focusing on issues that are most relevant to your own experience.

2. Find allies to support you. Family, friends, neighbors, and professionals all have roles to play. Your allies can support you, and help you work through the potential risks and benefits of the steps you include in your plan.

3. Find resources to work with. People can preserve their capacity to lead an ordinary, successful life. Institutions and systems offer access to treatment, and support the necessities of life. Groups like NAMI (the National Alliance on Mental Illness) and Mental Health America (formerly called the Mental Health Association) offer support, education and advocacy. Their members are familiar with the struggle.

4. Plan both near-term and long-term. The plans you make should always include meaningful human connection, as well as medical and legal advice from professionals you trust. Choose techniques that respect people, build on strengths, and increase independence.

5. Follow your plan. Take charge. Do what you need to do. Use your plan to guide your decisions. Revisit your plan when you get stuck or run into trouble. Do not fret if you are only partially successful. Everyone struggles with achieving success. Do not get discouraged. Action plans never play out as first written. Everyone is a work in progress.

THE COMMON STARTING POINT

Recovery is like a long journey on foot. Travel happens close to the ground. Terrain matters. Time matters. A trusted guide is essential. Even so, travelers are willing to start if the goal is important. The journey itself has value.

The starting point of a mental health recovery journey is like walking away from an accident, surviving a disaster, or arriving at a place that has been wiped out. A person might be stunned and shaky, and might need to figure out what to do, but the time to take action is at hand.

Thinking has been affected. Trauma, medical issues, and adverse life events cause people to lose "executive function," the ability to make plans or take action when there are no clear guidelines.

Feelings are affected. Shame, fear, sadness, loneliness, and anger must be expressed, worked through, and processed, not repressed.

Relationships are critical, but may need to be rebuilt. This is unavoidable tough work.

Information is missing. Time and technology move forward when people are stuck in troubled circumstances.

People at the starting point need allies. Friends and family can help keep people grounded in reality. They can help their friends practice thinking. They can help their friends work through the emotional effects of shame and trauma. They can help locate information, and facilitate access to services, and act as advocates when trouble is at hand.

DEFENSES AND DENIALS

It is hard to commit to recovery. People stay attached to habits, places, situations, and relationships that might not be good for them. On top of that, everyone uses a standard set of defenses and denials, what the author Mary Pipher calls "defenses against too much reality."

- We deny reality entirely.

- We accept some aspect of reality but deny other equally critical aspects.

- We minimize or normalize.

- We overemphasize our lack of power.

- We deny our emotional investment in reality.

- We compartmentalize.

- We feign apathy.

- We kill the messenger.

Even though we recognize that everyone avoids confronting something, postpones commitments, or has difficulty staying on a difficult path, we also know that people are not doomed to stay where they are stuck.

From childhood through adulthood, everyone has countless experiences of change. People confront their problems, try things, change what they are doing, learn what works, and complete hard tasks or completely transform themselves.

This often takes help, and the willingness to accept help.

TIMING ISSUES AND RESISTANCE

People frequently encounter awkward timing issues on the way to addressing a problem. When someone else is first to recognize a need to act, conflict ensues.

There is a pattern to committing to any behavior change or recovery journey, called stages of change. The most successful long-term path through timing and resistance issues often involves relationship building and collaboration, not control and coercion.

The first stage of the change process is pre-contemplation. At this point, the problem or difficulty does not even register on someone's personal radar. The task of helpers at this stage is to build or maintain a relationship, provide practical support, and look out for serious risk.

The second stage is contemplation and preparation, where a person starts to see a problem and develops the motivation to take action. Here the task of helpers is to maintain the relationship and help the person gather resolve.

The third stage is action. As a person starts addressing issues of concern, helpers maintain the relationship, accompany the person, and support progress.

The final stage is maintenance. As a person does what is required to support a stable life, helpers maintain the relationship and support the person's ongoing process.

Note that maintaining relationships is important throughout this change process. Relationships have power even when people are not thinking clearly. Potential helpers who want to learn more can consult Xavier Amador's book *I Am Not Sick I Don't Need Help!* or Milt Greek's book *Schizophrenia: A Blueprint for Recovery.* The Integrated Dual Diagnosis Treatment model for people with co-occurring mental health and substance abuse issues also stresses the power of collaborative relationships.

FAMILIES TRAVEL TOGETHER

Families often hold the key to accepting treatment and staying engaged in recovery. It is tough to maintain relationships when a person loses capacity due to illness. Everyone wants autonomy and has their own idea about what makes a good relationship. People resist dependency and too much support. Yet when someone we love is in genuine trouble, it is important to act.

Friends and family members often face the issue of their own capacity to be helpers. It may be challenging to maintain a relationship and live a normal family life, but there is more capacity within families than we might realize. Everyone wants health, safety, and success for the people closest to them. As a family confronts trouble, or someone in a family confronts a challenge, roles might change, but they need not become opposing roles. The point is to journey safely together.

GROWTH AND DEVELOPMENT SET THE CONTEXT

Much of what motivates people connects with the universal human experience. A human development perspective helps us understand our actions, desires, and experiences in the context of where we are in life. We can use this understanding to build motivation, promote learning, and achieve important goals.

People consciously or unconsciously try to create a path forward through life. We compare where we are with where we think we should be. If we listen to what people say about their life goals, we soon learn that nearly everybody yearns for normalcy and a good life. The presence or absence of a disability seldom affects this. Ask any young person with a disability what they want in life. What you will hear will sound amazingly normal. A boyfriend or girlfriend, a job, a family, more money, a better place to live. A future. These goals connect with a set of basic human desires and goals called the hierarchy of needs. People are motivated to satisfy all of these needs, but lower-level needs are so compelling that attaining one level actually frees up capacity to pay attention to higher-levels. Biological needs come first. Examples include food, sleep, and shelter. Safety needs come second. This category includes protection, stability, freedom from fear and anxiety, and need for rules in society. Love and belongingness are next. This category includes the need for family and friends, and the desire to avoid feelings of loneliness and isolation. Esteem needs follow. For example, we want favorable judgment from others as well as from ourselves. Self-actualization is the top level. Even if all the lower level needs are satisfied, we tend to feel unsatisfied unless we are doing all that we are capable of doing.

People also have an innate developmental agenda. We yearn to achieve what is normal for our stage of life. In early adulthood, people typically select mates, learn to live with a partner, start families, and start careers. By middle age, people expect to be in the midst of their careers, raising older children, or helping teenagers become adults. As people reach later maturity, they are adjusting to decreasing strength, finding appropriate living quarters, and building new relationships with others their age. The developmental tasks of adulthood can be a kind of positive benchmark that lets us shift our attention towards the kind of progress we might aim for.

A developmental lens changes how we view mental illness. Instead of tracking degrees of impairment, we can focus on what it takes to build or rebuild the capacity to achieve what we desire of life. Everyone is entitled to work towards achieving a meaningful, successful life.

The notion of recovery relates to where people think they need to be along life's path. Recovery is about maximizing the capacities and skills that are useful in making progress, while paying due regard to other critical issues such as health, safety and risk.

RECOVERY IS SOCIAL

Recovery from mental illness is a social process as well as a medical or psychological process. People are social creatures. We learn best through relationships. We create cultures, and adapt to the customs of the people around us. Only rarely does someone prosper alone. We live in families, learn in classes, work in groups, play team sports, and organize clubs and social events.

People with health issues often find that they must recover socially as well as clinically. There is practical value to companionship. Attending to social connections helps people make progress, and reduces the risk of tragic outcomes. Feelings of isolation and burden on others are linked closely to suicide.

Anyone can help or have a role to play in supporting recovery. Ordinary people help each other cope with depression, bipolar disorder, anxiety disorder, PTSD, and schizophrenia every single day in every culture on earth. Believing otherwise is a fantasy, a myth, an obstacle to the progress that we seek.

Support and compassion are valued by every culture, every religion. We may feel awkward around certain issues, but so what. Awkwardness sets the stage for bravery, grit, determination, and virtue. We can still commit to moving in a positive direction.

HOPE IS A PROCEDURE

Hope is a process everyone can access, with a toolkit that people already have. Hope is like empowerment. It starts out as a dream, and becomes real with action and practice. There is a process for gathering motivation, getting started, sticking with it, and addressing ongoing risk. Every single day, countless people of every skill level, every economic level, and every level of disease burden confront their challenges and make progress in their lives.

FOUR QUESTIONS FOR RECOVERY

Recovery is a process of building a person's capacity, empowering the person to overcome the effects of the illness. Every person has a range of talents and abilities, a variety of vulnerabilities, a certain capacity to withstand stress, and a certain risk of causing harm when something goes wrong.

Ask four questions to help build recovery.

1. What helps you make the most of your talents?

2. How can you reduce the areas where you are vulnerable?

3. How can you improve your ability to cope with stress?

4. How can you deal with the risk of something going wrong?

The answers will inform critical choices about treatment, medication, overall health, career, housing, and family relationships.

UNDERSTANDING RECOVERY

Successfully dealing with mental illness takes the right treatment, self-will/self-monitoring, family or community support or case management, vocational activity (including school), spirituality, and rediscovery and reconstruction of a sense of self.

We have all experienced recovery from a minor infection or an injury like a cut or sprain, but we also recognize that recovery from conditions like diabetes, asthma or arthritis is different. These are chronic illnesses, with symptoms that persist or flare up from time to time. Treatment might be essential, even if unpleasant. Chronic symptoms bring on fatigue or interfere with the tasks of daily life. All of us know people who accomplish important things despite the symptoms of their illness. We admire their courage, their character, and heart.

In the 1980s, a group of writers with mental illness began using the word recovery to describe their experience of coping with symptoms, getting the care they need, and regaining control of their lives. They described recovery as a process, an outlook, a vision, a guiding principle. Their main message was that hope is justified, and that restoration of a meaningful life is possible, even with a mental illness.

The early writings of the recovery movement were historic in one key sense: For the first time, people who experienced mental illness were expressing optimism about their hopes for a better, more fulfilling life, a life they could aspire to even though they continued to struggle.

Nowadays, these writings look like tentative first steps. They are not optimistic enough. We have learned that addressing mental health concerns is the path to more success. It is a sign of maturity. We have given up on making social outcasts of people who are working on their health issues. We view our communities as inclusive and pluralistic. We realize that people with health problems need support and care to regain capacity, stay connected to work, and restore relationships with friends and families. We cheer a good comeback, and applaud people who regain control of their lives. We recognize success, even when people struggle along the way.

There is still some tension between the medical model and the recovery model. The medical model focuses more on symptom relief, while the recovery model focuses on restoring self-esteem and identity. The recovery model does put more emphasis on what a person can achieve despite the persistence of symptoms. Despite these differences, there is a great deal of common ground. Reducing the symptoms of mental illness may be exactly what is needed to make progress possible.

BUILDING AND SUPPORTING RECOVERY

Learn what you can about the challenges that you are facing. This book is just a place to start. When using the Internet, look for sources that represent a mainstream consensus-based approach. Distinguish between the search for information and the experience of online socialization. Be wary of websites that push a certain product, and equally wary of websites that tell that you no product ever works. Do your research when things are going well. Do not wait for a crisis.

Recognize when symptoms are building up. Therapy helps people identify triggers and warning signs. Family and friends notice these patterns too. Create a game plan that addresses the buildup, the acute phase and the aftermath. Add strategies that relieve stress and help reduce symptoms. Write down when to call the doctor. Use the plan as a frame of reference when discussing events as they unfold. Discuss what happened and adjust the plan once a situation resolves.

Make informed decisions about medication and treatment. Always rely on medical advice. Do not stop taking medication on your own. A single person's feelings that a mental health condition is cured should probably not be trusted. If medication is hard to tolerate, call the doctor. If the doctor will not respond to these concerns, consider changing doctors.

Preserve family solidarity. Every family member reckons with the direct or indirect effects of the illness and deserves love and comfort. Keep communication going. Make sure everyone knows that their concerns are being heard. Talk about the struggle in inclusive terms. Plan together. Choose to identify strengths instead of assigning blame. Learn ways to handle conflict safely.

Learn how to recognize a person's capacity to function at the present moment. People benefit when they can act independently. A degree of support may sometimes allow a person to maintain control and achieve what they consider important. On the other hand, when the person is experiencing greater capacity, the same supports can restrict freedom and frustrate progress.

One function of an ally is to help with reality testing. Another is to support good communications. If someone is describing an ongoing hallucination, point out simply that you are not experiencing the hallucination. Do not pretend to believe or agree with delusional thinking. Respond to the emotional content (frustration, fear, anxiety). Memory loss or inability to concentrate can be extremely frustrating and frightening. Do not insist that the person with symptoms try harder to concentrate. Instead, find a place with fewer distractions. Repeat information calmly, in a nonjudgmental way.

Everyday tasks take longer when people lose capacity under stress. Build more time into daily routines. Do not rush. Do not demand that a person with mental illness "pull himself together." Not being able to do this is part of the illness. Do not expect and insist that all peculiar behaviors be corrected at once. Focus on what is accomplished, not on what is not accomplished.

EXPECT TO RECOVER ONE DAY AT A TIME

Garth House describes his journey towards recovery.

> Two and a half years ago, when I was recovering from a very devastating and negative relapse that included hospitalization, I can remember how fleeting and brief were the periods of relief from depression and from an eclipse of peace of mind that was almost complete.
>
> How precious these few moments of relief were to me; how valued just for a few moments of inner peace. They always came as a surprise, perhaps when I was washing dishes after a meal, or climbing the fire escape to my apart-

ment when the beauty of the setting sun against the brick and the iron caught my attention and lifted me to a wider perspective that made my suffering seem small and insignificant.

As I slowly recovered from my relapse, I found more and more periods of peace and serenity as I grew in strength and healed from the devastation of my illness. My gratitude for my recovery informed everything. The simplest acts in the workplace became important achievements, and there was no lack of meaning and direction in my life.

I wish I could tell you that the state described above lasted and grew with me as I continued in my recovery. Unfortunately, what began to happen was that I started taking things for granted. I lost my focus on the day at hand, and consequently failed to live one day at a time. The joy and satisfaction I took from every action performed in the course of a day slowly faded away, and I began to place upon myself demands that were not reasonable and expectations that could not be met. As a consequence I began to become depressed. I struggled to find purpose.

I became ungrounded. I longed for those brief moments in my early recovery where everything was reconciled in peace.

Today I understand the importance of staying focused in the present moment. I look upon the work of recovery (at least part of it) to be a conscious, deliberate effort to remain positive and grateful for each moment of the day. It also helps me to remember just how much I have survived in my illness and to congratulate myself for all I have overcome.

It also helps me to realize that the challenge to live life on life's terms comes in three-fold form:

First, there is the illness to attend to. As a person with manic-depressive illness, I must understand that depression is a symptom. By naming this for what it is, I rob it of some of its power over me.

Second, reality, by its very nature, is full of ups and downs. There are moments of peace and moments of turmoil. All of us, with or without mental illness, must deal with this aspect of reality.

Third, to perceive the eternal beauty that rests in the present moment requires the discipline of a lifetime and is not come by cheaply. We who have walked the tortuous path of mental illness understand the simplest of beauty and the smallest pocket of serenity. This is both the gift of our illness and its greatest challenge.

FAMILIES LEARN TO COPE

Judy Thomas, a NAMI Ohio board member, discusses her story and her hopes for the future.

When your family member first becomes ill, no matter if it is sudden and traumatic, or it creeps up little by little until it cannot be denied, the world as you have known it will change. What do you do when your family member is diagnosed with a severe, persistent, long-term disease such as schizophrenia, bipolar illness or any one of a myriad of similar diseases?

Feelings and reactions may vary from family to family and individual to individual. Yet guilt, anger, fear, denial, grief and uncertainty as to what to do to help are probably universal to some degree. Grieving is real. You grieve "for the person who used to be," and for all their future promise which may be lost. Moving forward is painful and difficult. You will need to grieve the loss of your own expectations and then move on to support your family member. Finding a way to balance the responsibilities of everyday life with those of care for the ill person will test the fiber of the family unit. But families do learn to cope and they do survive. It is done every day-one day at a time.

To elaborate, families may feel a whole range of emotions. Confusion and disorientation. Denial and distancing, expressed as "This can't be happening to me." Guilt based on several misconceptions, including "I should have recognized this sooner," or "I'm the parent, I must be to blame." Fear of the stigma of mental illness. Fear for the safety of the ill person and sometimes for the safety of others. Anger over serious difficulties in trying to get help for the ill person. Anger toward professionals because the family is excluded from treatment decisions. Extreme fatigue caused by trauma of events. And desire to escape from "the nightmare."

You need to give yourself and your family time to process and understand the changes that have occurred. The experiences you have had with other illnesses in the past will be of little help. Educate yourself concerning every aspect of the illness; it will bring you compassion and help to dissipate some of the anger. Find a support system as soon as you possibly can. Your local NAMI group will contain people who share your feelings and are in various stages of experience with mental illness. The NAMI Family-To-Family Program will provide you with education about mental illness, medications, and how to find help.

When you are ready I strongly advise you to take this course.

Families have a role and a place in the treatment process. Know that your family member's past medical and personal history and your insights and perspectives are needed, especially in the beginning, when the person is very ill and may not be able to communicate with health professionals. Treatment and rehabilitation services are provided in the community, but there are major gaps in the mental health system. People depend on family and friends for help and support. It takes determination to battle mental illness. A new life must be built. New structures for daily living must be developed.

A supportive and caring family helps in the recovery process, but, at the same time, you must care for yourself. Maintain your independent life and identity and resist becoming consumed by the illness. Continue to develop your own interests.

Always hope for healing. The medications do work and new ones are being developed all the time. Brain research and development of new medications without the difficult side effects of older drugs will change the face of mental illness in the future, so never lose hope.

CONFRONTING THE CHALLENGE OF STIGMA

Stigma surrounds mental illness, and taints most everything connected with it. Advocacy groups and people with mental illness have been working to wipe out this stigma for decades. Progress is slow. Stigma connects with social distancing, a process that starts in infancy that helps us learn who is safe and who might be dangerous. Because it is part of an innate human process, stigma is difficult to displace.

Stigma is grounded in fear. Author Pete Earley describes the cruel mechanics of stigma in his 2006 book *Crazy*, which examines how police, courts, and jails deal with people with mental illness.

> We lock up the mentally ill because they terrify us. We are afraid of them and even more frightened of what they symbolize. We want to believe they did something that caused their insanity. That is why we can justify housing them in inhumane conditions and punishing rather than treating them. The federal government says mental illness is a chemical imbalance, and because of that it's a sickness and not something... that anyone seeks or wants or deserves to get any more than he seeks, wants, or deserves to get a cold.

> But deep down, we really don't want to believe that's true. Because if we did, we would have to admit: *It could happen to us. It could happen to me...* And

that is such a frightening thought that we quietly search for explanations to prove that the mentally ill aren't like us and they somehow deserve the torment they suffer.

The stigma of mental illness, together with the devastating effects these illnesses can have on people's lives, also makes for conflict and controversy. Passions run high because the stakes can be so high.

Reciting brain facts to indifferent audiences will not end stigma. Mental illness stigma persists even after decades of well-meant educational campaigns. A better path starts with person-to-person connections, and disclosure.

Whether or not to disclose a history of mental illness is always a tough choice, but the experience of Betty Ford and others in eliminating the former stigma surrounding breast cancer offers hope that wiping out the stigma of mental illness is possible.

Widespread disclosure would be a step towards creating a more inclusive, diverse, polycentric, successful society. We are safer and healthier without self-inflicted blind spots. We can learn to see our strengths, reckon with our limits, and help each other make progress.

HOW TO USE THIS BOOK

Defying Mental Illness is designed to help people solve problems. How to understand what someone is experiencing. How to recover. How to help a friend or neighbor. The whole text is a summary of what people contend with, and what helps people make progress. Use the Table of Contents or the search function in your ebook reader to locate specific topics.

Part One is a basic guide to mental health disorders and treatment, a brief survey of what people are facing. For people who are not clinicians, mental illness is not that complicated. The basic patterns take a short time to explain.

Part Two is about allies. This part of the book shows how people with symptoms, the treatment team, family members, friends, and community members can align their efforts. Everyone has a role in supporting and promoting good health.

Part Three covers resource issues, including health insurance, housing, employment, and disability benefits.

Part Four is about safety and risk. Topics include mental breakdowns, suicide, violence, criminal justice, involuntary hospitalization, and guardianship. These issues often require acting on two overlapping timelines, one that addresses immediate needs, and another that builds long-term progress.

Part Five is about creating a plan and taking action. A person's strengths, interests, and capacities are the seeds of a positive future.

The *Defying Mental Illness* website **www.defyingmentalillness.net** contains downloadable worksheets, videos, and links to additional resources.

PART ONE
FACING MENTAL ILLNESS

MENTAL ILLNESS FACT BOOK

Mental illness has a significant impact on the United States economy and on the nation's overall health. Mental illness is at the root of many issues encountered in the criminal justice system. It connects to poverty, homelessness, substance abuse and sometimes contributes to violence.

Mental disorders are the leading cause of disability in North America. Four of the ten leading causes of disability in the U.S. and other developed countries are mental disorders. Some 90 percent of the 38,000 suicides occurring each year in the United States connect with mental illness. Suicide is the third leading cause of death among young people aged 15-24. The disease burden of mental illness, including suicide, is second only to cardiovascular disease. Cancer is third.

The economic impact of not treating mental illness is greater than the cost of treatment. The cost of untreated mental illness impacts the economy in the form of lost productivity, absenteeism and increased medical expenses.

The treatment success rate for mental illness can be up to 80 percent. One in 10 Americans experiences a mental health disorder serious enough to affect work, school, or family life every year. Less than half get help.

COMMON FEATURES

Authors John Ratey and Catherine Johnson compare mental illness to persistent unacceptable levels of mental noise.

> While most of us will never hear voices, all of us have had the experience of being blasted by sounds and stimuli we cannot block out. We know how disorienting noise can be. We even have an expression for how we feel when the world is too loud: We say we "can't hear ourselves think."

Everything about the experience of mental illness is a matter of degrees. Ordinary aspects of our lives help us relate to what people with mental illness are experiencing. None of us is immune from trouble. Everyone experiences a full range of emotions. We know sadness, excitement, and anxiety. We lose focus, get confused, feel lonely, and regret things we did when we were angry. Sometimes we don't feel anything. We become fascinated by some things, and lose interest in others. We get suspicious and avoid bad news. We appreciate moments of solitude. Everyone refuses to believe something that other people swear by. Some of us even hear voices.

The term "mental illness" is used to describe behavior, thoughts, or feelings that go far beyond the normal range of experience. Mental illness is disabling, distressing, and persists for substantial periods of time. It involves severe disturbances in thinking, feeling, and relating, as well as difficulty coping with the ordinary demands of life.

It is important to understand that mental illness is biological. It is not a person's fault or a moral failure. Mental illness is a medical issue related to how a person's brain is functioning. Biological processes are impacting the person's thoughts, capacities, and emotions. These processes are rooted in evolution and genetics, and are connected to every experience the person has had in life. On top of that, improving brain function is a complicated proposition. The human brain is the most complex biological structure we know of. It is controlled by an extremely complex mix of chemical and electrical processes affected by the many functions of the body. Because our brains are highly complex and dynamic, and constantly changing, it should not surprise us that some things might go wrong, and that fixing these things will not be simple.

Fortunately, we do not need a graduate course in brain biology to recognize symptoms of mental illness. Even though every person's experience of symptoms is different, certain patterns of behavior, thinking and emotional experience do emerge. Diagnostic labels are simply names for these patterns. Researchers have correlated some of the patterns to what they observe in brain biology, but the science is not yet exact. To a certain extent, diagnostic labels are also social-historical constructs. Certain diagnoses seem to come in and out of fashion. In addition, there is a range to this. Mental illness is often a matter of degrees, not an on-off proposition.

Mental illness makes us reflect about variety and diversity. People have so many kinds of strengths. Everyone is different. We know that every person retains some abilities even when other capacities are lost, uncontrolled, or distorted. We should question where to draw the line with medicalizing the human condition. Our world benefits from a diversity of experience and interests and talents. We do not want every distressing human experience labeled as some type of sickness. Still, at some point there is just too much. At some point, as a person loses capacity to function in the world, the only prudent course is to do what we must to make things better or keep people safe.

People with mental illness all experience at least some of the thoughts, feelings, and behaviors listed in the catalog of typical symptoms and behaviors that appears below. A single symptom or isolated event is not usually a sign of mental illness. Multiple, severe or sustained episodes that interfere with the ordinary processes of life do need to be addressed.

The symptoms of mental illness come and go in cycles, and vary in severity from time to time. The duration of an episode also varies. Some people are affected for a few weeks or months, while others experience the illness for many years or for a lifetime. There may be no reliable way to predict the course of a person's illness. Symptoms may change from year to year, and differ from person to person even with the same diagnosis. Many people have combinations of problems (called co-occurring disorders) that interact in complex ways.

Stress makes symptoms worse. Anyone can lose sleep, become anxious, and lose effectiveness or even collapse ("break down") or act out under too much stress. This passes quickly for most people. However, when people with chronic mental health conditions experience stress, they have much more symptom burden, and much more trouble maintaining self-control. They are much more likely to act impulsively and cause harm or get into trouble with the law.

CATALOG OF TYPICAL SYMPTOMS AND BEHAVIORS

CHANGES IN THINKING OR PERCEIVING

- Hallucinations
- Delusions
- Excessive fears or suspiciousness
- Inability to concentrate

CHANGES IN MOOD

- Sadness coming out of nowhere, unrelated to events or circumstances
- Extreme excitement or euphoria
- Pessimism, perceiving the world as gray and lifeless
- Expressions of hopelessness
- Loss of interest in once pleasurable activities
- Thinking or talking about suicide

CHANGES IN BEHAVIOR

- Sitting and doing nothing
- Friendlessness

- Abnormal self-involvement
- Dropping out of activities
- Decline in academic or athletic performance
- Hostility, from one formerly pleasant and friendly
- Indifference, even in highly important situations
- Inability to express joy
- Inappropriate laughter
- Inability to concentrate or cope with minor problems
- Irrational statements
- Peculiar use of words or language structure
- Involvement in automobile accidents
- Drug or alcohol abuse
- Forgetfulness and loss of valuable possessions
- Attempts to escape through geographic change
- Frequent moves or hitchhiking trips
- Bizarre behavior (skipping, staring, strange posturing)
- Unusual sensitivity to noises, light, clothing

PHYSICAL CHANGES

- Hyperactivity or inactivity (sometimes alternating)
- Deterioration in hygiene or personal care
- Unexplained weight gain or loss

- Sleeping too much or being unable to sleep

REACHING A DIAGNOSIS

Because the brain is so complex, and because mental illness is expressed through behavior, diagnosing mental illness is not easy.

A thorough physical examination is usually the first step in figuring out what is wrong. Diseases such as hypothyroidism, multiple sclerosis, or a brain tumor can cause many symptoms that look like mental illness. Unfortunately, physical measurements like blood tests seldom reveal quick answers.

People seeking help are engaged in conversation and are asked a series of questions. Information from relatives, friends, and employers about the person's behavior also helps with the diagnosis process.

The diagnosis process involves comparing descriptions of a person's behavior and feelings to listings in a catalog of disorders called the DSM (Diagnostic and Statistical Manual). The diagnosis is merely a label in a classification system. There are just a few major classifications, but each has sublistings, variations in severity, duration and other features. The DSM authors aim for consensus, but there will always be some uncertainty in classification systems when the subject matter is so complex. The latest revision of the DSM was criticized for both increasing the number of diagnostic labels, and for eliminating others. Because nonclinicians do not diagnose anybody, there is seldom any benefit to over-focusing on the DSM's technicalities or even its various flaws.

It is not unusual for a person's stated diagnostic label to change over time.

SCHIZOPHRENIA

Schizophrenia affects thinking and judgment, sensory perception, and the ability to appropriately interpret and respond to situations or stimuli. Schizophrenia does not mean that someone has more than one distinct personality. Although the word schizophrenia does come from a Greek term meaning "splitting of the mind," the notion that someone with schizophrenia has a "split personality" or "dual personality" is incorrect.

People with schizophrenia have "positive symptoms" (hallucinations or delusions), "negative symptoms" (apathy, loss of connection to other people), and cognitive symptoms (thought processing problems). Hallucinations involve hearing, feeling, or seeing things that exist only in the mind of the individual. Delusions are persistent false beliefs. Psychosis means that severe hallucinations or delusions are disconnecting the person from the common experience of reality. People with schizophrenia experience suspiciousness, withdrawal, communication difficulties, and drastic changes in behavior and personality.

There is a tremendous range to what people with schizophrenia might experience. Even when a person's experience of symptoms is severe, the person retains many capacities and talents.

People with schizophrenia discern meaning from experiences that reflect both ordinary reality and their hallucinations or delusions. This can result in poor insight (the inability to recognize that one is ill), an especially difficult symptom. Poor insight may persist even when other symptoms such as hallucinations and delusions respond to treatment. This lack of insight is more extreme than the type of resistance or denial we all experience when something in our lives might need attention or change. People must essentially learn their way out of lack of insight. This is a long-term proposition requiring significant trust-building work and support from family members, friends, and treatment professionals.

People can develop schizophrenia at any age. The onset of the first psychotic episode usually occurs around 21 years of age for men and 26 years of age for women. When the disease first appears, people feel tense and develop an inability to concentrate or sleep. They begin to withdraw. Their schoolwork (if they are still in high school or college) may deteriorate. Their general appearance may worsen. Their friends may drift away. Parents sometimes think that it is just adolescent behavior gone astray. Sometimes doctors use a tentative diagnosis in the early stages. It may take several psychotic episodes to reach a definite diagnosis.

People may be reluctant to tell others about their symptoms. The symptoms of schizophrenia frighten people. Paranoia is especially terrifying. Some people do not realize that their experience differs from how other people perceive the world. They may assume that other people hear voices, too.

Many symptoms of schizophrenia involve increases or decreases in activity, emotion, or thinking processes. Pay attention to the velocity and direction of change. People develop symptom patterns that can help predict when they will need help.

Alterations of the senses. People experience intensified sensations (typically early in the disease), or blunted sensations (usually later in the course of the illness).

Inability to synthesize and respond. People with schizophrenia have trouble filtering out information, deciding what is relevant, putting ideas together, and figuring out what to do. Disruptions in processing thoughts and emotions can make people feel "disconnected" from the world. The ability to test logical connections becomes impaired. Cause and effect relationships become distorted. Independent events become symbolically connected. Speech patterns change. People with schizophrenia may speak in specifics rather than generalities and with excessive levels of detail (called concreteness), or use made-up words (neologisms), or speak with confused strings of repetitious words that seem to make no sense (schizophasia or "word salad").

Delusions and hallucinations. Hallucinations are sensory perceptions with no external stimuli. People with schizophrenia most often "hear voices." Delusions are beliefs not based in reality and usually connect to inappropriate associations or logic patterns within the person's thinking. Delusions can be very elaborate. People with paranoid delusions believe they are being watched or persecuted. People with grandiose delusions think that they are wealthy, or have special powers, or that they are famous. People with religious delusions believe they receive special messages from God or have divine powers or a divine identity. Many people experiencing delusions claim their thoughts are radiating out of their head and being broadcast over radio or TV.

Altered sense of self. People with this symptom experience confusion with respect to where their body ends and the external world begins.

Changes in emotions. Emotions intensify or become very restricted. People experience widely varying and rapidly fluctuating emotions and exaggerated feelings, and may talk of guilt or fear. Or they may experience flattened emotions, which appear as apathy, slowness of movement, underactivity, and lack of drive.

Changes in behavior. People with schizophrenia may withdraw from others, remaining quietly in one place for long periods, sometimes even becoming immobile. Some people develop ritualistic movements or patterns of behavior.

Schizophrenia originates from very complex interactions among genetic factors, environmental factors (including trauma), fetal development, brain structure, and brain functioning. There is no cure for schizophrenia. Many medications can reduce symptoms. Finding the right medication(s) is a very complex process that requires a trusting and working relationship between the person with the symptoms and the doctor. Every medication causes side effects. Make sure to discuss the impact of the medication on overall health. Occasionally, symptoms disappear on their own.

People with schizophrenia benefit from medical treatment, but also need understanding, compassion, respect, and motivation to pursue recovery. People with severe symptoms may need help with the activities of daily life. Community support programs (case management programs) can connect clients with services and help with finding housing and other essentials.

Family life can be more beneficial than any social service program, especially when focused on inclusion and support. Parents and family should not blame themselves for the onset of this illness. Families do need to come to terms with the emotions surrounding the illness. It is important to be as supportive as possible. It is especially important to recognize and foster the skills and talents that the person retains. Stress makes it harder to control symptoms.

Most people achieve their recovery goals. Symptoms abate just enough, although they may re-emerge from time to time. Many people with schizophrenia enjoy success in life. They stay connected with their families. They find or retain employment, and have careers.

THE EXPERIENCE OF SCHIZOPHRENIA

Many people with schizophrenia experience auditory hallucinations. The voices they hear are intrusive and unpleasant. The author Lori Schiller describes hearing voices at age 17 at summer camp.

> Then, in the middle of this chaos, a huge Voice boomed out through the darkness.
>
> "You must die!"

> Other Voices joined in. "You must die! You will die!"

> At first I didn't realize where I was...But as soon as I realized that I was in my bunk, and awake, and that my roommate was still sleeping peacefully, I knew I had to run. I had to get away from those terrible, evil Voices. I leaped from my bed and ran barefoot out into the grass.

Milt Greek describes hallucinations as "waking dreams."

> Hallucinatory reality is analogous to dreaming in the same room where a television is on. The physical reality of the television is translated into the idiosyncratic symbols of the person's dreaming and the person's consciousness experiences the dream, not the television.

MOOD DISORDERS

Bipolar disorder (also known as manic-depressive illness) and major depression are "affective" disorders or mood disorders. Profound changes in emotions can be accompanied by physical ("somatic") effects.

BIPOLAR DISORDER (MANIC-DEPRESSIVE ILLNESS)

In bipolar disorder, also known as manic-depressive illness, the individual swings between periods of depression ("low" mood) and periods of mania, a persistent, excessively "high" or "irritable" mood. People usually experience periods of normal moods in between these two "poles." Some people experience "rapid cycling," where mood swings rapidly back and forth between depression and mania with no stable periods in between. People can also experience mania and depression at the same time.

There are several variations of bipolar disorder. Some people do not experience full-blown mania, but experience a less extreme form of mania called hypomania. This condition is called "bipolar II disorder." People with bipolar II disorder are frequently misdiagnosed as having major depression. This is because hypomania feels normal and highly productive, and people are more likely to look for help when they cycle into depression. If misdiagnosed, a person risks being prescribed antidepressant medication without mood-stabilizing medication. This can push a person with bipolar II disorder into full-blown mania.

Bipolar disorder and major depression tend to run in families. If both parents have bipolar illness, their children have a 75 percent chance of having some form of mood disorder.

Bipolar illness sometimes appears in childhood or adolescence. The majority of cases begin in young adulthood. It almost never develops after the age of 35.

Mania refers to extremely elevated mood, often with irritability, hyperactivity, and decreased need for sleep, and sometimes including delusions and paranoia. Since some of these symptoms also occur in schizophrenia, it is difficult to diagnose which illness an individual has. Some of the symptoms of mania can lead people to believe that they are not sick. In fact, they assert that they have never felt better. The euphoric mood may continue even in the face of sad or tragic situations. The person may go days at a time without sleep, and does not even feel tired.

Although the person may feel euphoric and think nothing is wrong, family and friends may notice serious problems. People with mania go on spending sprees, become promiscuous, drive recklessly, or abuse drugs and alcohol without realizing that these behaviors are abnormal. Irritability can bring on extremely abusive verbal outbursts, which the person with the illness believes are justified.

Fortunately, bipolar disorder is very treatable. Lithium carbonate, a mood stabilizer, is effective for 70 percent of people with bipolar disorder. It completely eliminates symptoms for one out of five people and substantially reduces symptoms for the others. Lithium also has a protective effect for people at risk for suicide. Many other medications are also available. Newer medications may not be any more effective than older types of medication. Every medication has side effects. When considering any medication, make sure to discuss the impact of the medication on the person's overall health.

People with bipolar disorder must learn to recognize their moods and implement strategies that head off problems. Psychotherapy, especially cognitive-behavioral therapy, and support groups help people come to terms with their illness and achieve recovery.

THE EXPERIENCE OF BIPOLAR DISORDER

Kay Redfield Jamison, a clinical psychologist on the staff of Johns Hopkins University Medical School, describes her personal experience of manic-depressive illness.

> There is a particular kind of pain, elation, loneliness and terror involved in this kind of madness. When you're high it's tremendous. The ideas and feelings are fast and frequent like shooting stars and you follow them until you find better and brighter ones. Shyness goes, the right words and gestures are suddenly there, the power to seduce and captivate others a felt certainty. There are interests found in uninteresting people. Sensuality is pervasive and the desire to seduce and be seduced irresistible. Feelings of ease, intensity, power, well-being, financial omnipotence, and euphoria now pervade one's marrow.

> Somewhere, this changes. The fast ideas are too fast and there are far too many; overwhelming confusion replaces clarity. Memory goes. Humor and absorption on friends' faces are replaced by fear and concern. Everything previously moving with the grain is now against — you are irritable, angry, frightened, uncontrollable, and enmeshed totally in the blackest caves of the mind. You never knew those caves were there. It will never end.

Madness carves its own reality: It goes on and on and finally there are only others' recollections of your behavior — bizarre, frenetic, aimless behaviors — for mania has some grace in at least partially obliterating memories.

What then, after the medications, psychiatrist, despair, depression and overdose? All those incredible feelings to sort through. Who is being too polite to say what? Who knows what? What did I do? Why? And most hauntingly, when will it happen again?

MAJOR DEPRESSION

Everyone experiences feelings of sadness or being "blue," but major depression is much more sustained, disabling, and severe. Major depression has a visceral impact, sometimes even physical symptoms. People with severe depression find they cannot work or participate in daily activities, and frequently feel that death would be preferable to a life of such pain. Depression is linked to suicide.

Depression is a very common illness, affecting as many of twenty percent of women and ten percent of men at least once in their lifetimes. Depression can appear at any age. Depression is very common among children and adolescents, as well as among older adults. Some people have severe, recurrent depression, with episodes as frequently as once or twice a year. Episodes of depression may last six months or more.

Many women experience "postpartum depression" after giving birth. Do not ignore postpartum depression. It can lead to severe disruptions in family life and potentially tragic outcomes.

Do not ignore or downplay symptoms of depression. Seek professional help promptly. Tell your doctor what you are experiencing. Go through your entire list of symptoms. Disclose any thoughts you have had about suicide.

Key symptoms of depression include feelings of sadness, hopelessness, guilt, or worthlessness. Inability to concentrate. Loss of energy. Changes in eating or sleeping habits. Most people with depression will have difficulty sleeping, and may awaken one or two hours earlier than planned. Others will have difficulty staying awake and may sleep too much. Most people with depression will have decreased appetite and may lose a great deal of weight while others may gain weight. Depression can also cause physical symptoms, called somatic symptoms, involving aches, pains, headaches, or worse.

Anxiety frequently accompanies depression.

There are many types of depression. Searching for the "psychological cause" may or may not help. Although depression can resolve on its own, effective treatment can reduce the length of episodes and the severity of symptoms. Each person responds differently to antidepressant medications and psychotherapy. It may take time to find the right treatment, even though many medications and therapies have similar rates of effectiveness. Exercise can also help with depression.

To a greater or lesser extent, everyone with depression carries on and copes as best as they can, even with ongoing symptoms. The struggle involves doing whatever it takes to stay connected with work and family life until depression lifts, and to recruit allies who can help head off danger.

The most effective course of treatment combines psychotherapy and medication. Access to treatment varies. In the U.S. a person's health insurance coverage determines the type and quality of the options available. Many people are never referred to a psychiatrist. General practitioners prescribe most of the antidepressant medications used in the U.S.

Until recently, medication for depression consisted of several groups of drugs classified as "antidepressants." In recent years, certain medications originally developed as antipsychotic agents for treating schizophrenia have been approved for use in treating depression, especially "treatment resistant" types of depression. This does not mean that antipsychotic medication works better than traditional types of antidepressant medication for most people, or that these medications are appropriate for most people seeking help. Most antidepressants (and several forms of psychotherapy) have about the same rate of effectiveness. The differences from the point of view of the patient mostly relate to price, risk of toxicity, and side effects. When discussing medication, make sure to discuss the impact of the medication on overall health.

Closely monitor people taking antidepressant medication. The risk of suicide increases as the person becomes more "activated" following a period of deep depression.

Probably more than with any other illness, people with depression are blamed for their problems and are told to snap out of it, or pull themselves together. People may even be told they have no right to be depressed. It is critical for family and friends to understand that depression is a serious illness. People cannot snap out of serious illness. Imagine telling someone to snap out of heart disease or cancer.

Do not underestimate the benefit of love and support from friends and family. People who are depressed need to hear that they are loved, valued, and connected to others, and that any feelings of worthlessness or abandonment the person may have are mistaken.

THE EXPERIENCE OF MAJOR DEPRESSION

The author William Styron describes his experience with depression in his 1990 book *Darkness Visible, a Memoir of Madness.*

> The madness of depression is, generally speaking, the antithesis of violence. It is a storm indeed, but a storm of murk. Soon evident are the slowed-down responses, near paralysis, psychic energy throttled back close to zero. Ultimately, the body is affected and feels sapped, drained.
>
> That fall, as the disorder gradually took full possession of my system, I began to conceive that my mind itself was like

one of those outmoded small-town telephone exchanges, being gradually inundated by floodwaters: one by one, the normal circuits began to drown, causing some of the functions of the body and nearly all of those of instinct and intellect to slowly disconnect.

There is a well-known checklist of some of these functions and their failures. Mine conked out fairly close to schedule, many of them following the pattern of depressive seizures. I particularly remember the lamentable near disappearance of my voice... The libido also made an early exit, as it does in most illnesses — it is the superfluous need of a body in beleaguered emergency. Many people lose all appetite; mine was relatively normal, but I found myself eating only for subsistence: food, like everything else within the scope of sensation, was utterly without savor. Most distressing of all the instinctual disruptions was that of sleep, along with a complete absence of dreams.

Exhaustion combined with sleeplessness is a rare torture.

SCHIZOAFFECTIVE DISORDER

Schizoaffective disorder combines psychotic symptoms such as hallucinations or delusions with significant mood symptoms of depression or mania. People with this disorder are likely to have symptoms that shift over time, showing more or less of the mood or psychotic symptoms at various points. Schizoaffective disorder is less common than either schizophrenia or bipolar disorder. It affects more women than men. The average age of onset is later than that of schizophrenia, usually in the late 20s.

ANXIETY DISORDERS

Anxiety disorders include panic disorder, posttraumatic stress disorder (PTSD), and obsessive-compulsive disorder (OCD). People with many other mental health conditions frequently have additional symptoms of one or more anxiety disorders.

In their milder forms, anxiety disorders are the most common psychiatric disorders. When more severe, these disorders can be extremely disabling.

Cognitive-behavioral therapy, sometimes combined with medication, is the usual way of treating anxiety disorders. This type of therapy combines discussions of a person's recurring thought patterns with carefully structured "real-world" experiences.

PANIC DISORDER

In panic disorder, people have repeated "panic attacks" that come "out of the blue" when there is nothing to fear. These include symptoms such as sweating, shortness of breath, heart palpitations, choking, and faintness. The person may be convinced that he or she is having a heart attack or is going to die.

POST-TRAUMATIC STRESS DISORDER

Post-traumatic stress disorder (PTSD) results from exposure to a traumatic event. Trauma and stress can have lasting physical and psychological effects and may also affect a person's behavior. Cascades of hormones that are part of the immediate "fight or flight" response also prime a person for future action. Sometimes the person stays stuck on high alert. Overwhelming stress or repeated exposure to stress can leave the person anxious and depressed.

PTSD becomes self-reinforcing. People with PTSD have been primed to re-experience the traumatic event. They relive or replay the event in their memories or dreams. Even when awake, shock or stress could trigger the sensation that the traumatic event is happening again. The fight or flight response kicks in once more.

Symptoms of PTSD include avoidance of certain stimuli, feelings of detachment or numbing, sleep disturbance, angry outbursts, concentration and memory problems, hypervigilance, and exaggerated startle response. People with PTSD may abuse alcohol or drugs to alleviate these symptoms.

Trauma in childhood can lead to difficulties in managing emotions, difficulties with executive function (the ability to decide on a course of action when a path is not clear), and difficulties in school. Childhood trauma also connects with future criminal behavior and addiction. Combat trauma can disrupt the lives of military veterans returning to their families and communities. Trauma is common among people involved with the criminal justice system, and among people with substance abuse problems.

For many people, healing begins once someone asks, "What happened to you?" instead of "What's wrong with you?"

Treatment involves talk therapy, sometimes with medication. Therapy helps people learn skills to overcome destructive thought patterns, and rebuilds capacity to encounter situations they have been avoiding. People who experienced childhood trauma learn to reframe their experiences and recognize their personal strengths.

THE EXPERIENCE OF POST-TRAUMATIC STRESS DISORDER

Blogger Caroline Spring writes about how she experiences the recurring effects of trauma.

> And then there are the times when I am assaulted on every side by flashbacks and somatic symptoms, that barrage of body memories that crashes relentlessly into my body and mind: nausea, headaches, grey pain and sharp pain, earaches, fever, exhaustion, insomnia. It's as if your whole body is mashed up with malfunction. So crisis doesn't take just one form. But at the core of each of these clusters of symptoms is a sense of overwhelming panic, of powerlessness and loss of control, of the unbearability of emotions, and a cloistering, febrile sense of self-hatred which fuels me towards self-destruction.

OBSESSIVE-COMPULSIVE DISORDER

Obsessive-compulsive disorder (OCD) is very common. Many people have slight cases that hardly interfere at all with daily life. Others have severe symptoms that make it difficult to function effectively in the world. Obsessions are repeated, intrusive, unwanted thoughts that cause extreme anxiety. Compulsions are ritual behaviors that diminish anxiety. Common examples are hand washing, counting, checking (to see if the door is locked or the coffeepot turned off, for example), and repeating (a word or action). Some people have only obsessions and some have only compulsions, but most people with obsessive-compulsive disorder have both. Stress makes symptoms worse.

BORDERLINE PERSONALITY DISORDER

Borderline Personality Disorder (BPD) is a serious, potentially life-threatening disorder characterized by severe emotional pain and difficulty managing emotions. People with BPD experience severe negative emotions like anger, shame, and fear of abandonment and have extremely volatile moods. They have difficulty maintaining a stable and accepting sense of self. They act impulsively, often negatively, striking out and harming loved ones or themselves. Family and social relationships are chaotic. Employment, long-term planning, and relationships can be severely impaired.

People with borderline personality disorder are at high risk of suicide. The suicide rate of people with borderline personality disorder is more than 50 times higher than the rate of the general population. Many people with borderline personality disorder attempt suicide multiple times.

Treatment for borderline personality disorder usually includes both psychotherapy and medication. Medication can help reduce anxiety, depression, and disruptive impulses. This can help the person engage in therapy and make progress. Clinicians work diligently to sustain relationships with their patients who have borderline personality disorder. They handle decisions about medication collaboratively, and take into account the person's willingness to take the medication, the side effect profile of the medication, and particularly the risk of overdose.

EATING DISORDERS

Eating is never simple. Within an instant of our first breath, eating takes hold of our whole bodies, a warm, embracing combination of sight, touch, thought, taste, smell, sensation, and emotion. Eating builds our first relationships, and continues as a source of social and cultural experience. We alter our diets in order to express our values or religious commitment, or to communicate our independence, social standing, or adventurousness. Eating may fade into the background of our lives, but never stops being essential to life, and never loses its intimate connection to emotion and memory.

We are used to casually saying that people in the midst of an eating disorder are trying to imitate culturally promoted, idealized body types, but that is an oversimplification. Eating disorders start with behavior that serves a conscious or unconscious purpose. There may be some sensitivity or vulnerability, or perhaps some event, trauma, or family dysfunction that the person must process. Some 40 to 60 percent of people who come to therapy for an eating problem have experienced physical or sexual abuse. Some abuse survivors are actually trying to render themselves unattractive, to de-sexualize themselves to prevent future abuse, while others are striving to become "perfect." People with eating disorders might also be reacting to bullying, or experiencing other sorts of issues that have affected their ability to maintain healthy psychological boundaries. For example, they might have had important aspects of their lives over-controlled (or grossly undercontrolled) during childhood.

Trauma, boundary issues, and emotion-driven eating all connect with secrecy. People often find a way to move forward with their lives once they deal with the secrets they have been carrying.

When people have idealized a certain body type, or misperceive their own, they must, to a certain extent, learn their way back to health.

EATING DISORDER TYPES

People with eating disorders are dealing with much more than a simple failure to achieve a healthy weight. These disorders involve constant concern about food or weight, and behaviors that are extreme or threaten the physical processes of the body. Treatment can become an urgent matter, and often involves medical supervision plus attention to thoughts and emotions.

Anorexia nervosa is maintaining a starvation diet. **Bulimia nervosa** involves cycles of binge eating and purging (forced vomiting, use of diuretics or laxatives, or drowning the body through excessive fluid intake), and can sometimes involve restrictive eating and excessive exercise. People with bulimia may even have a normal body weight. **Binge eating** involves large quantities of food, and is the most common eating disorder. **Pica** involves eating substances that are not food. There is also a catch-all category called **Eating Disorder, Not Otherwise Specified**.

Ninety percent of people with anorexia or bulimia are women. Men experience eating disorders too. About forty percent of people with binge eating disorder are men. Eating disorders usually show up in the teenage years, but can arise earlier or later in life.

Eating disorders have the highest death rate of any psychological disorder. Some effects accumulate over the long term. Others are medical emergencies that can happen at any time. Purging causes electrolyte imbalances that can lead to heart attacks or strokes. Dehydration can lead to heart failure or death. Malnutrition can result in respiratory infections, kidney failure, blindness, heart attack, and death. People who binge on fluids (more than eight eight-ounce glasses of water in a day) can lose their capacity to regulate sodium, which may cause fluid to accumulate in the lungs, plus brain swelling, nausea, vomiting, extreme confusion, even death.

Beyond the physical effects, people with eating disorders can experience disordered thinking and great emotional distress. Imagine experiencing a negative body image, an addiction, a mood disorder, and an anxiety disorder all heaped together.

Many people with eating disorders engage in non-lethal self-harming behaviors like hitting, scratching, cutting, or burning themselves.

Suicide is another danger. People with anorexia or bulimia have a suicide mortality rate 23 times higher than that of the general population.

WARNING SIGNS

- Eating disorder warning signs tend to accumulate around a person.

- An obsession with weight or food.

- Knowing exactly how many calories or grams of fat are in food items, and obsessively pointing it out.

- A need to exercise all the time.

- Avoiding hanging out with friends during meals.

- Wearing baggy clothes, hiding their shape.

- Dramatic or very restrictive diets.

- Cutting up food into tiny pieces, rearranging items on the plate without eating them.

- Competing with others about how little they eat.

- Going to the bathroom a lot, especially right after meals.

- Talking about being fat despite losing a lot of weight.

- Being defensive or sensitive about weight loss or eating habits.

- Buying or taking laxatives, steroids, or diet pills.

- Not menstruating or infrequently menstruating.

- Having a tendency to faint.

- Bruising easily.

- Having very pale skin.

- Being cold or complaining of being cold.

These are just some of the most common symptoms a friend or family member might notice. There are many other signals. A young person's friends may be the first to notice what is happening. Sometimes there are clues in social media postings.

Anyone who notices these indicators piling up should talk to the person about their concerns, and, if possible, accompany the person to see a counselor or medical person, or even a parent to start getting help. Unfortunately, resistance and denial are common. After all, everyone finds it hard to come to terms with having a problem.

It is important that that the person hears that friends will stay supportive no matter what.

Should someone refuse an offer of help, it is important to take action anyway. Friends should share their worries with an adult who can take the next step towards assessing the situation, such as a school counselor, the person's parent, even a hotline. The National Eating Disorders Association has an information and referral service at 1-800-931-2237.

TREATMENT AND RECOVERY

Treatment starts with a visit to a doctor or an emergency room for a medical exam, blood tests, and an interview. People need appropriate initial medical treatment, plus diligent attention to a recovery process, and ongoing social support. The treatment team helps the person recalibrate their self-image, and helps them safely process any trauma that has caused them harm.

Inpatient programs resemble addiction treatment centers, with medical monitoring plus therapy plus cooking class. Especially at first, people require sufficient monitoring and supervision to prevent old habits from reemerging. Supervision lessens as people make progress. Relapse is common, so people learn what to do when it occurs. Recovery and relapse prevention build the capacity to lead a balanced, positive life.

Many people recover from eating disorders and enjoy healthy lives. Many young women from the fashion industry, the entertainment industry, dance, and athletics have revealed their experiences of eating disorders. They attribute their long-term success to skills they learned in recovery.

SUBSTANCE ABUSE, ADDICTION, AND RECOVERY

The danger and suffering surrounding addiction, as well as the transformative nature of the recovery experience, tend to attract drama and dogmatism. If you or your family are confronting an addiction issue, it helps to filter out the drama and tune down the dogmatism – with one exception: If you are working a recovery program, stick with what is helping you.

Addiction and recovery are biopsychosocial issues. After a certain point, substance use (or any behavior capable of becoming a habit) changes brain function, changes thinking, and changes interactions with others. These changes can be long-term or permanent. People continue their habits despite the consequences they experience. Anyone can become addicted, and anyone who manages to achieve sobriety must work hard to maintain it. Relapse is a constant threat.

The biological effects of addiction can start with the first dose. The drugs people abuse are often toxic, delivering their effects by impairing some aspect of the body's function. Toxicity, plus the state of the user's health, plus the other circumstances around the use of the drug, can make any dose of a toxic substance a fatal dose. Another toxic risk factor is increased tolerance. Over time, as the body adapts, it takes more of the substance or activity to deliver an effect. A person with a high tolerance may survive drug exposures that would kill someone else. Many fatalities are linked to changes in drug tolerance. If a person loses drug tolerance, a regular dose becomes a fatal dose. Risk multiplies when people combine drugs, or drink alcohol while using drugs. Every drug can cause health consequences, and beyond the drug's direct effects, the circumstances under which people take drugs increase infectious disease risk. Infectious diseases connected with injection use include infective endocarditis (a heart infection), HIV, and Hepatitis B and C.

Psychological and social effects are long lasting. Addiction hijacks brain capacities, resulting in cognitive distortions, disregard for safety, and disregard for others. As cravings reorient a person's life to repeating the experience of the drug or the habit, personal and social consequences pile up. People lose employment, build up debt, lose custody of their children, commit crimes, and incur criminal penalties. Destroyed relationships, delinquent child support obligations, tax consequences, probation requirements, and restitution orders are common.

Even when people experiencing addiction sincerely desire to stop their drug use or end their distressing behavior, they find this extraordinarily difficult to accomplish. Withdrawal can be painful, even dangerous. Even if a substance has no specific physiological withdrawal effects, addiction's cognitive effects undermine efforts to change. This is why recovery from addiction requires more than detox, more than willpower. Recovery must go further and deeper. It takes a sustained combination process of personal action, culture change, and social support to restore brain function. Quite naturally, people who have achieved recovery often become committed advocates for the program that worked for them.

Before the invention of Alcoholics Anonymous (AA) in the 1930s, few people ever recovered from alcoholism or addiction. There were no effective clinical models. Alcoholism and addiction were relentless unstoppable processes that led to social isolation, impoverishment, medical complications, and death. Bill Wilson, who invented AA, noticed that the few people who recovered often did so through religious conversion. Wilson developed AA as an experience of group process, step progression, periodic rewards, recognition, mentoring, and self-study, very similar to methods religious groups have used for centuries to initiate members and sustain their communities. A person who works the AA process achieves sobriety with enough support to sustain long-term recovery.

AA helps perhaps one out of every three or four individuals who attempt it. Other nonclinical approaches to recovery complement the work of AA. They serve people who have difficulty relating to AA concepts. Women for Sobriety dispenses with the notion of powerlessness, but retains a fair amount of other AA content. LifeRing considers recovery to be the result of the person's own motivation and effort. The group has meetings and online sessions that support abstinence, but no "step program" and no religious content. SMART Recovery is cognitive, secular, and strength-based. It uses a workbook of cognitive retraining exercises plus recovery group meetings to promote and support long-term abstinence. Rational Recovery is a non-group methodology.

All nonclinical support groups use simple published texts (or programs) designed for general audiences. In AA and other nonclinical support groups, meetings are led by people who have experienced addiction themselves ("peers"), not by clinicians.

The dominant model of clinical addiction treatment in the US is the so-called Minnesota Model, essentially AA adapted for institutional settings. People are hospitalized in secure units, supervised through a short detoxification process, followed by an inpatient or residential experience, followed by extended stays in smaller community facilities (halfway houses), or in homes or apartments shared with other people in recovery (sober living). People who live in the community may attend full day or half-day intensive outpatient programs of individual psychotherapy, group therapy, or education sessions, plus AA or other recovery group meetings. Length of treatment is important. The longer a person stays in treatment, the more likely the person will remain free of relapse.

In clinical settings, treatment targets the person's individual situation, and involves a variety of well-documented individual and group therapy techniques. Counselors, clinical social workers, or other professionals lead the sessions. Because addiction and recovery are biological processes, medication can also play a role. Unfortunately, no medication wipes out addiction. Medication substitutes for drugs that are more dangerous. It helps people manage withdrawal symptoms, or addresses co-occurring health issues such as mental health disorders. Medications used as substitutes for street drugs are often addictive themselves. Good programs track medication use and ensure that medication is not diverted to the street drug trade. Medication increases program retention, reduces drug-seeking behavior, reduces injection-related infections, and lowers overdose death rates.

DRUGS OF ABUSE

Caution: Detailed information about drugs of abuse is beyond the scope of this book. In an emergency, dial 1-800-222-1222 to reach the Poison Center that serves you. Your call will be routed to the Poison Center that serves your area. A good starting point for reference purposes is the National Institute on Drug Abuse website, www.drugabuse.gov.

Any drug can be abused. Many of the drugs listed below have valid medical applications. Unfortunately, misuse of prescription drugs has become a major health threat. More people are dying in the United States from prescription drugs than from heroin and cocaine combined. Deaths involving prescription pills quadrupled between 1999 and 2010. About 6.1 million people abuse prescription pills. Overdose deaths have at least doubled in 29 states, where they now exceed vehicle-related deaths. In 10 of those states, rates tripled. In four of them, they quadrupled.

Tobacco contains nicotine, a stimulant that increases blood pressure and heart rate. Tobacco causes numerous types of cancer, inhibits lung function, causes heart disease, and causes birth defects. Tobacco is highly addictive. Tobacco-related illnesses are among the most common causes of death for people with mental illness. Americans with mental illnesses have a 70 percent greater likelihood of smoking than the general population. Because tobacco use can be one of the first negative "boundary crossing" activities among young people, tobacco use at a young age may indicate problems to come.

Alcohol is the single most abused drug in the United States. In low doses, alcohol provides mild stimulation and a sense of euphoria, but in higher doses alcohol is a depressant. Alcohol lowers inhibitions, lowers response times, and dramatically increases risk of injury, violence, and suicide. Alcohol use during pregnancy can harm the fetus, and is the most common cause of intellectual disability (formerly known as mental retardation). Alcohol poisoning can be fatal. Because withdrawal from alcohol can be fatal, alcohol detox must always be supervised. Alcohol dramatically increases the fatal overdose risk of other drugs.

Opiates reduce pain, slow reactions, and produce euphoria. Drugs in this category include opium, morphine, heroin, oxycodone, hydrocodone, codeine, fentanyl, methadone, and others. Health risks include slow or arrested breathing, lowered pulse and blood pressure, unconsciousness, coma, and death. These drugs have significant fatal overdose risk. Fatal overdose risk skyrockets when opiates are combined with alcohol use. **Opiate overdose rescue kits.** The drug naloxone can interrupt or reverse opiate overdoses. The drug is packaged as a nasal spray for first aid kits. Naloxone puts a person into immediate opiate withdrawal by displacing opiates from the body's receptors. This restores central nervous system function and respiration. Urgent medical attention is still required. Unfortunately, naloxone is not available for first aid in many states.

Depressants slow metabolism, reduce anxiety, and create a calming effect. Drugs in this category include barbiturates (Amytal, Nembutal, Seconal, Phenobarbital), benzodiazepines (Ativan, Halcyon, Librium, Valium, Xanax, Klonopin), and sleep medications (Ambien, Sonata, Lunesta). Health risks include slowed pulse, lowered blood pressure, and slowed breathing. Drinking alcohol with any of these drugs increases the risk of respiratory failure and death. Withdrawal from barbiturates can be life threatening.

Stimulants increase alertness, movement speed, and thought processes. Drugs in this category include amphetamines (Biphetamine, Dexedrine, and Adderall), methylphenadate (Ritalin, Concerta), cocaine, and methamphetamine. Health effects include increased heart rate, increased blood pressure, panic, paranoia, violent behavior, psychosis, weight loss, and insomnia. Snorting cocaine causes nasal damage. Methamphetamine causes severe dental problems. **Bath salts** are stimulants made with an assortment of chemicals that can cause heart palpitations, kidney failure, liver failure, behavior changes, suicidal thoughts, aggression, and violence.

Hallucinogens cause changes in perception, thought and consciousness. Drugs in this category include LSD, mescaline, and psilocybin. Health effects include increased body temperature, increased heart rate, tremors, numbness, memory loss, impulsive behavior. LSD can cause flashbacks and persistent hallucinations.

Cannabinoids cause euphoria and relaxation. Drugs in this category include marijuana, hashish, and THC. Health effects include slowed reaction time, distorted sensory perception, impaired balance and coordination, increased heart rate and appetite, impaired learning, impaired memory, panic attacks, psychosis, frequent respiratory infections, and possible mental health decline.

So-called **club drugs** tend to be distributed at nightclubs, concerts, and social events. Ecstasy (MDMA) has mild hallucinogenic effects and lowers inhibition, but also causes anxiety, chills, sweating, cramping, sleep disturbances, and depression. Rohypnol and GHB cause drowsiness, sedation, memory impairment, and blackouts.

Anabolic steroids are used to "bulk up" or improve athletic performance. They do not produce intoxication effects. These drugs cause hypertension, liver cysts, hostility, aggression, and premature growth stoppage. They have various sex-specific effects: Among males, these drugs cause prostate cancer, reduced sperm production, shrunken testicles, and breast enlargement. Among females, these drugs cause menstrual irregularities and development of masculine characteristics.

Inhalants such as solvents, paint thinner, glue, or gases produce intoxication, stimulation, loss of inhibition, loss of motor coordination, and other effects. Inhalants damage the cardiovascular system and the nervous system. They can cause memory loss, loss of consciousness, and sudden death.

STARTING ADDICTION RECOVERY

All that is needed to begin addiction recovery is a starting place and a way to move forward. The starting place is not defined by the amount of suffering that precedes it. People should not use the concept of "hitting bottom" as an excuse to continue with their addiction. Follow the basic strategy: Find out what you are facing – this section of the book is enough to start with. The next step is to find allies. The way to move forward can be a call to a doctor, a visit to a clinic, a conversation with a pastor, or even typing AA or the name of another recovery program in an internet search box. Nonclinical resources can support a person waiting for clinical resources to open up. The recovery community can help identify a path forward, and can support a person through the journey.

Family members must have their own recovery. At a minimum they must learn how to maintain the relationship with the person, while refusing to support the addictive behavior. Sometimes the family must step up and take action to protect a person whose life is in danger. The process to compel addiction or mental health treatment varies from state to state. This may be lifesaving.

CO-OCCURRING MENTAL ILLNESS AND ADDICTION

People with mental illness have a greater chance of becoming abusers of alcohol or illicit drugs than do members of the general population.

People with mental illness frequently turn to alcohol or drugs to try to escape from their symptoms. More than half of all people with a substance abuse problem have some type of mental illness. The incidence of schizophrenia among people with substance abuse problems is almost four times the rate of schizophrenia in the general population. The incidence of serious mood disorders among people with a substance abuse diagnosis is over five times that of people in the general population.

There is a clear connection between childhood mental illness and substance abuse later in life. Children with mental health issues at age 8 may start using alcohol or other drugs a few years later, many times before age 12.

People with both mental illness and a substance abuse disorder are said to have "co-occurring disorders" or "dual diagnosis." People with co-occurring disorders experience more severe and chronic medical, social, and emotional problems compared to people with a mental health issue alone. They are more vulnerable to alcohol or drug relapse, which worsens the psychiatric disorder. They require longer treatment, proceed more gradually in treatment, and experience crisis more frequently. They are far more prone to violence than people who do not abuse drugs or alcohol. They require customized relapse prevention training because standard relapse prevention techniques do not work effectively for them.

Mental illness and addiction have many features in common. They are biological illnesses, hereditary at least in part, chronic and incurable. They lead to lack of control of behavior and emotions. They have positive symptoms (added but unwanted behaviors) and negative symptoms (loss of ordinary functions of life). They affect the entire family. They get worse if not treated. They can be controlled with the proper treatment. They are diseases of denial, causing feelings of guilt and failure. Both mental illness and addiction are stigmatized, improperly judged moral issues caused by personal weakness, rather than disorders with a biological basis. Recognizing that one has mental illness or an addiction can lead to depression and despair.

Stigma interferes with treatment of these conditions. Even when people do enter treatment, they frequently try to conceal one or another of these issues. When someone begins a treatment program for either substance abuse or mental illness, the family or friends should make sure that the treatment team learns about any accompanying mental illness or substance abuse problems.

Despite the common features of mental illness and addiction, their respective treatment systems are quite different. Mental illness and substance abuse treatment systems developed along different historical paths. They are controlled by separate statutes and separate funding streams. They have separate regulatory and credentialing systems. The philosophies and cultures of the two systems conflict. The addictions system emphasizes peer counseling, spiritual recovery, self-help, confrontation, detachment, and empowerment. The mental health system emphasizes treatment by medical professionals, scientific treatment, medication, support services, case management, and supervision. The messages to the person in recovery conflict.

When the two systems do not collaborate, people receiving treatment for co-occurring disorders are prone to abandon treatment and relapse. The most effective treatment model for people with co-occurring disorders is integrated treatment. This represents more than the person being treated for two conditions by two separate agencies at once. Integrated care means everyone works together from a single unified treatment plan.

HOW TREATMENT WORKS

Mental illnesses are biological disorders of the brain. The human brain is hugely complicated, with billions of connections between nerve cells. Everyone's brain changes over the course of a lifetime. Everything — genetic factors, the course of development prior to birth, the experiences of childhood, nutritional choices, health and disease, experience of love and affection or of stress and trauma, physical injury — in fact nearly everything in our background and experience has a subtle physical expression in the brain. This characteristic is called plasticity.

A human brain operates with cascades of extremely complicated chemical and electrical signals. The brain relies on chemical substances called neurotransmitters to carry signals from one brain cell (called a neuron) to another. The part of a neuron that receives the chemical signals is called a receptor. Each receptor is tuned to receive a certain type of chemical signal. The nature and intensity of the signal received determines the signals each neuron sends down the line, and the pathway each signal takes within the brain. These signals generate further responses within the brain and throughout the body. Experiences generate new connections between neurons, or strengthen existing connections, while other connections become disused or lost.

The brain's plasticity explains how psychotherapy works and how medication works. Because the brain changes physically with experience, the experience of talking through, thinking through, and resolving problems has the potential of making the needed changes in brain functioning. Medications directly affect brain function by manipulating the chemical neurotransmitter mix, or by altering the effectiveness of the receptors, thus changing the brain's capacity to use certain neurotransmitters. Other non-medication techniques, like those involving magnetic fields, also work by altering the dynamic patterns of brain function.

Every technique used to improve brain function is imprecise. Recovery takes time and effort, and a willingness to learn what works.

CONVERSATION AS THERAPY

People throughout history and in every culture have met with one another to talk through problems. Talking through problems with family, friends, clergy, or professionals has helped resolve countless difficulties and personal issues through the ages. Conversations can be powerful. They can actually change brain function. It is not an instantaneous process. Working things out takes work. However, if you really succeed in changing your way of thinking, you have in fact changed your brain!

Psychotherapy turns conversation into mental health treatment. There are many different types of psychotherapy. Examples include psychoanalytic psychotherapy, cognitive-behavioral therapy, group therapy, motivational therapy, and family therapy. Every licensed therapist is schooled in a variety of therapy techniques. These techniques are studied and evaluated, just like medication. They have histories, instruction manuals and bodies of literature that are accessible to people making decisions about treatment.

Because psychotherapy is medical treatment, therapists are subject to state laws and codes of ethics. These rules govern important issues such as proper conduct for the therapist, treatment confidentiality, and disclosure of information. Matters discussed in therapy are confidential, with some limits and exceptions. The most critical exceptions to confidentiality include threatened harm to self or others, and abuse of a child or other vulnerable person. Therapists keep their clients well informed about the rules governing confidentiality.

The relationship between client and therapist is one of the keys to effective therapy. The client must feel safe within the therapeutic setting, because therapeutic conversations sometimes involve painful, secret thoughts and feelings.

Because confidentiality is so important to preserving the therapeutic relationship, the other people helping a psychotherapy patient can sometimes feel they are being "shut out." When proper consent is in place, caregivers of people in therapy can gain access to some information about therapy sessions. However, even signed consent forms rarely produce more than summary reports about the effects of therapy.

Most therapists will accept information from family members about issues facing the person in treatment. However, because of the extremely private, sensitive nature of therapy, most "outsiders" still find themselves wanting more information than the therapist is willing to share.

TREATMENT WITH MEDICATION

Note: The main groups of psychotropic medications are discussed below. This information is a summary, intended for general educational purposes only. It does not substitute for a physician's advice.

Mental illnesses are like any other medical condition. Some people require medication to treat their illness effectively. Although some people benefit from talk therapy alone, many others require medication or a combination of medication and psychotherapy to relieve their symptoms.

Studies documenting the long-term effectiveness of various treatments for mental illness are accessible on medical reference websites.

Psychotropic medications (psychiatric drugs) can help people think more clearly, and can help people gain control of their thoughts and actions. Medications can help bring emotions back within a normal range.

The beneficial effects of many medications may not become noticeable for several weeks. The maximum beneficial effect may take months of continuous use to develop.

It is risky to discontinue medication without a doctor's supervision. Medication may take days or weeks for the body to process and for effects to wear off. People who stop taking medication may not see their symptoms return immediately. Symptoms controlled by the medication return some time later. The risk of symptoms returning escalates after medication stops. The consequences can be life threatening for many people.

Medications are potent, but no medication works for every individual. Expect prescriptions to change over time. Experience with one class of medication can sometimes predict the probability of success with another, but it is difficult to know exactly how much benefit a person will obtain from a particular medication, or the type and severity of the side effects that the person will experience. Most people change medications from time to time. A course of medication that has helped someone for months or years may lose effectiveness for that individual. In addition, members of different ethnic groups metabolize certain medications differently and may require adjusted dosages.

Any licensed physician can prescribe psychotropic medication. Many primary care doctors are quite experienced with common medication issues relating to depression, attention deficit disorder, or anxiety. Psychiatrists specialize in the treatment of mental illness. People may see one doctor for medication management, and a separate clinician for talk therapy.

Medical supervision is especially important for people at risk for suicide. People who start on antidepressant medication have increased risk for suicide when they start becoming more activated.

Psychotropic medications produce both beneficial effects and undesirable effects (side effects). Each medication has its own side effect profile. Side effects of psychotropic medications can occur early in therapy or may not appear until after months, or occasionally years, of use. Some side effects, especially many that appear early, are temporary and may go away or become less severe after a few weeks. Most side effects relate to dosage. The higher the dose, the worse the side effect. Some medications can cause long-lasting side effects that persist well after discontinuing the medication. Unfortunately, some side effects are permanent, even fatal.

UNDERSTANDING INFORMED CHOICE

Everyone who begins any form of treatment is entitled to an informed choice. This means that a person fully understands all the arguments, all the costs and benefits of all available options, before making a choice. This is a matter of medical ethics and human rights.

Treatment should proceed within a framework of person-centered, strength-based care. Medical team members usually have more technical knowledge than the person who is making the choice, but should act more as teachers or counselors than as people in positions of power or control. Unfortunately, in the field of mental health, this standard has been easy to violate. People arrive in great distress for scarce appointments with medical personnel who may be perpetuating social distance and stigma. Medical providers might feel entitled to exercise power because they have hard-earned expertise. In today's pressured healthcare environment people tend to push things along. This happens even when the provider's duty is to slow down and take the time needed to communicate options and ensure that they are being understood.

In the US, with very few exceptions, members of the medical team may not initiate treatment without a person's permission. When a person loses capacity due to illness, and cannot make an informed choice, a substitute decision-maker (such as a guardian or conservator) has a duty to consider the wishes and best interests of the person, and make an informed choice in the person's stead. When a person is involuntarily committed to a hospital, the court supervises the medical team.

Every person in treatment is entitled to choose the goals of treatment and to know what to expect from any proposed treatment. People are entitled to know the risks and benefits of medications, including the potential long-term effects of the medication on overall health. Cost is important too. Newer, more expensive medications may provide essentially the same benefit as older or generic medications. On the other hand, a newer medication could be the absolute best overall choice.

Proper dosage is also important. Unfortunately, some physicians prescribe too much medication, to the point that treatment itself becomes uncomfortable or even disabling. People stop taking medication when this happens, and may lose confidence in treatment. Contact the doctor if medication is hard to tolerate. A lower dose may leave a person with some mental health symptoms, but restore enough capacity for the person to feel more in control of life.

Do not hesitate to become better informed about any course of treatment. Medications have been developed and used over the course of decades. An entire body of literature recounts people's experience with psychotropic medication. Internet resources are plentiful, but vary in quality.

Ethics issues do occur from time to time. Pharmaceutical manufacturers use a variety of marketing and advertising material to influence medication sales. Some physicians and hospitals receive substantial fees for product studies or for making presentations about products they prescribe. Many public mental health systems rely on product donations or discounts from manufacturers. Manufacturer incentives may or may not be voluntarily disclosed to patients.

Overmedication of people who depend on others for care may be interpreted as abuse or neglect.

Be especially careful of risk when considering experimental treatment.

KEY MEDICATION CONCERNS

Weight gain, hyperglycemia (high blood sugar) and diabetes rank among the most serious long-term health consequences of psychiatric medication. Physical health conditions account for the majority of the premature deaths among people with schizophrenia, bipolar disorder, and major depression. People with schizophrenia, bipolar disorder, and major depression have rates of cardiovascular disease, diabetes, respiratory disease and infectious diseases that are several times greater than the general population. Do not underestimate this type of risk. Although these health effects can be somewhat controlled with proper physical health care, proper diet, and exercise, it is extremely difficult for people with severe mental illness to achieve an optimal, healthy lifestyle. Many people without mental illness symptoms struggle unsuccessfully with obesity, lack of exercise and poor nutrition. On the other hand, some people with mental illness do substantially increase vigorous exercise or implement comprehensive dietary change.

Always review the information provided by the manufacturer or pharmacy regarding effective dosage, therapeutic effect, side effects, drug interactions, and special risks associated with specific medications. Check independent news and reference sources too. Because some people respond differently to medications from different manufacturers, you should note both the trade and generic names of the medications as well as the response and any side effects. Trade names of drugs are usually capitalized. Generic names usually appear in lower case.

People taking psychotropic medication should keep a written record of the name, dosage, and dates of use of each medication. This may be very important information to have later. Be sure that doctors, dentists, and pharmacists are kept informed of all medications that a person takes. This includes over-the-counter medications, vitamins, and nutritional supplements. Keep everyone involved in treatment informed about any known allergies.

Do not focus your attention narrowly on medication. Many people do recover from their symptoms and live without any medication at all, or learn to accommodate a certain level of symptoms and lead a normal life, but this rarely happens without support and appropriate medical advice. A course of psychotherapy and some follow-up may be enough for some people. Sometimes a combination of diet and exercise helps relieve symptoms to the point where medication is no longer necessary.

Coming to terms with what must be done to recover from serious illness is never easy. It is hard to accept a permanent dependence on medication with tough side effects. Very few of us scrupulously follow every instruction we receive about any medication. We have all postponed doctor visits, discontinued treatment, or failed to comply with instructions on a label. Nearly everyone tries to discontinue medication at some point. Remain calm if you learn that someone has discontinued taking medication. Doctors usually advise reducing doses slowly over a period of weeks. They closely monitor what their patients are experiencing. Treat this situation as an opportunity to be supportive, and to see what is necessary for a person's success.

Some people do need to take medication regularly in order to protect themselves or others from harm. Legal standards for involuntary administration of medication vary from state to state. Forcing someone to take medication is limited to extreme situations, usually involving serious, immediate risk of harm to self or others. When a person cannot live safely without medication or other treatment, a guardianship or conservatorship may prove necessary. This difficult step may be a person's only path to safety.

FIRST-GENERATION ANTIPSYCHOTIC MEDICATIONS

The first-generation ("traditional") antipsychotic medications have been used for well over half a century.

The main use of this group of medications is to counteract the "positive symptoms" of psychotic disorders, primarily schizophrenia. Positive symptoms are symptoms that "add to" normal behaviors. These include hallucinations, delusions, agitation, bizarre mannerisms, and disturbed thought processes. These medications do not affect the "negative" symptoms of psychotic disorders. Negative symptoms are those that "subtract from" ordinary behavior. Negative symptoms include withdrawal and apathy.

First-generation antipsychotic medications are also sometimes used to calm the severely hyperactive behavior seen in the manic phase of manic-depressive illness (bipolar disorder).

First-generation antipsychotic medications include chlorpromazine (Thorazine), thioridazine (Mellaril), mesoridazine (Serentil), trifluoperazaine (Stelazine), perphenazine (Trilafon), fluphenazine (Prolixin), thiothixine (Navane), chloroprothixine (Taractan), loxapine (Loxitane), haloperidol (Haldol), and molindone (Moban).

Haldol and Prolixin can be administered by injection at intervals of one, two, or several weeks. This eliminates the need to take the medication daily and can be useful when people tend to forget to take their medication or refuse to take medication, but is at high risk of harm without it.

Unpleasant side effects are common with these medications. People often refuse to take antipsychotic medication because of the side effects. Take complaints about side effects seriously, and bring them to the attention of the case manager/physician.

Some important side effects of this group of medications include:

Allergic reactions. If these occur, it is usually in the first two months of treatment. Notify the physician if any of these symptoms occur: yellowish skin, skin rash, flu-like symptoms such as fever, sore throat, stomach or intestinal pain or tenderness, vomiting, and/or diarrhea.

Autonomic reactions. These are reactions having to do with central "automatic" functioning of the body, such as salivary gland secretion, control of the heart and the circulatory system, digestive function, function of the eye, and numerous others. These usually appear early in treatment and may decrease or disappear after a few weeks. The most common are dizziness or even fainting when first sitting or standing up after lying down, dry mouth, blurred vision, difficulty in urinating, and constipation.

Drowsiness. This can be strong at first but may decrease or disappear after a few weeks of treatment.

Movement problems. There are several types of movement problems. Most can be treated by reducing the dose of antipsychotic medications or by adding other medications to counteract the problem. Movement problems usually appear within the first three months of treatment. Mild to severe muscle spasms may appear within the first few days of treatment. Some people experience **akathisia**, a sense of internal tension along with an inability to stay still (pacing, foot tapping, rocking, etc.). Some side effects mimic Parkinson's disease. These include tremors, shuffling gait, muscle stiffness, slow movement, and drooling.

Tardive dyskinesia. Mouth or facial effects including tongue protrusion, chewing movements, lip smacking, grimacing, or frowning are usually seen only after long-term use. Early signs of tardive dyskinesia should be reported to the physician promptly. Unless the medication is changed or the dose reduced, the symptoms may get worse and/or become irreversible.

ATYPICAL ANTIPSYCHOTIC MEDICATIONS

The second-generation ("atypical") antipsychotic medications work somewhat differently than the older "traditional" antipsychotic medications. Atypical antipsychotics control both the "positive" symptoms of schizophrenia (hallucinations and delusions) and the "negative" symptoms such as apathy and social withdrawal.

Unfortunately, these medications have at times been marketed as though they were highly benign and free of side effects, particularly when compared to the first-generation antipsychotics. Such assertions have proven to be over-optimistic. Some of these claims have even been litigated. People may still encounter these marketing claims from time to time.

Medications in this category include clozapine (Clozaril), risperidone (Risperdal), olanzapine (Zyprexa), quetiapine fumarate (Seroquel), ziprasidone (Geodon), and aripiprazole (Abilify).

Each atypical antipsychotic medication has its own side effect profile. Side effects of atypical antipsychotics also vary from person to person, by dosage, and by duration of use. Pay close attention to the warning labels.

Side effects of atypical antipsychotic medications include the following:

Weight gain, hyperglycemia (high blood sugar) and diabetes are among the most serious long-term consequences of use of these medications.

Tardive dyskinesia. Mouth or facial effects including tongue protrusion, chewing movements, lip smacking, grimacing, or frowning are usually seen only after long-term use. Early signs of tardive dyskinesia should be reported to the physician promptly. Unless the medication is changed or the dose reduced, the symptoms may get worse and/or become irreversible. Tardive dyskinesia is usually seen only after long-term use, sometimes only after decades of use. Atypical antipsychotics have not been used for that long, so the true risk of tardive dyskinesia is not known yet. All the atypical antipsychotics carry warnings about the possibility of tardive dyskinesia in their package inserts and in the Physician's Desk Reference (PDR). Early signs of tardive dyskinesia should be reported to the physician promptly. Unless the medication is changed or the dose reduced, the symptoms may get worse and/or become irreversible.

Akathisia is a sense of internal tension along with an inability to stay still (pacing, foot tapping, rocking, etc.).

Shifts in sleep patterns may occur.

Extreme tiredness and weakness are common with several of these medications.

Sexual dysfunction may be a side effect of psychotropic medication or a symptom of the underlying mental health condition.

Some medications require periodic testing and follow-up to guard against known risks. Clozapine (Clozaril) is one example. Clozapine can be effective for a substantial number of people who do not respond to other antipsychotic medications. However, Clozapine can be dangerous, and must be taken with caution. People taking clozapine can develop agranulocytosis (loss of white blood cells) that can be fatal if not recognized and treated early. To be safe, people taking clozapine require weekly or biweekly white blood cell testing. Seizures have also been reported by individuals taking clozapine. The medication is still useful for many people, but the risks must be taken into account, and proper precautions must be in place.

ANTIDEPRESSANT MEDICATIONS

Antidepressant medications are mainly used to treat depression. However, some of them are also used to treat anxiety disorders such as panic disorder and obsessive-compulsive disorder.

These drugs relieve depressed moods. They do not work by making the person intoxicated or "high."

People should be monitored closely when they are being prescribed antidepressant medication. Antidepressants are activating agents. When the depression starts lifting, a person may still be experiencing severe distress or agitation, but may become able to summon the effort to take destructive actions that were impossible before. Many antidepressants carry warnings about an increased risk of suicide. Some people with bipolar disorder can be pushed into manic states when taking an antidepressant without other mood stabilizing medication.

Antidepressant medications have been prescribed for decades. Studies concerning their effectiveness, and accounts of the experience of people taking the medication, are readily available.

Antidepressant medications are usually divided into four groups, each having different side effects.

Serotonin-selective reuptake inhibitors (SSRIs) include fluoxetine (Prozac), sertraline (Zoloft), and paroxetine (Paxil). The more frequent side effects are nausea, diarrhea, headache, hand tremor, nervousness, and insomnia. These medications are less dangerous when taken in overdose than some other classes of antidepressant medication.

Tricyclic antidepressants and related agents include imipramine (Tofranil), disipramine (Norpramin), trimipramine (Surmontil), amitriptyline (Elavil), nortriptyline (Pamelor), protriptyline (Vivactil), doxepine (Adapin, Sinequan), amoxapine (Asendin), and maprotiline (Ludiomil). Side effects include autonomic reactions, which are reactions having to do with central "automatic" functioning of the body, such as salivary gland secretion, control of the heart and the circulatory system, digestive function, function of the eye, and numerous others. The most common autonomic reactions are dizziness or even fainting when first sitting or standing up after lying down, dry mouth, blurred vision, difficulty in urinating, and constipation. People taking tricyclic antidepressants also may experience drowsiness and fatigue, which may decrease with continued use. These medications can also cause increased seizures in people with a seizure disorder and worsened heart disease in people with cardiac conditions. Tricyclic antidepressants are quite toxic. Overdoses are potentially fatal. It is important to follow the prescribed dosage.

Monoamine oxidase inhibitors (MAOIs) include tranylcypromine (Parnate), phenelzine (Nardil), and isocarboxazid (Marplan). A major problem with monoamine oxidase inhibitors is that people taking them must avoid certain foods (red wine, chocolate and many others) and certain prescription and nonprescription medications. Failure to avoid these items can result in a very serious or even fatal reaction. A list of foods and medications to avoid will be provided by physician and pharmacists. The more common side effects of these medications are dizziness or fainting when first sitting or standing up after lying down, restlessness, insomnia, and weight gain. Like the tricyclic antidepressants, the monoamine oxidase inhibitors are quite toxic. Overdoses are potentially fatal.

Miscellaneous agents include bupropion (Wellbutrin), trazodone (Desyrel), nefatodone (Serzone), and venlafaxine (Effexor). The most common side effects of bupropion are nausea, constipation, headache, hand tremor, dry mouth, nervousness, and insomnia. A significant problem with bupropion is its tendency to cause seizures, particularly when given in high dosage or to people with a seizure disorder. Trazodone's most frequent side effects are strong drowsiness, dry mouth, and dizziness when first sitting or standing up after lying down. Nefatodone is similar to trazodone, but may produce less intense side effects. Venlafaxine has a side effect profile that resembles that of the SSRIs, although it is not a true SSRI agent.

MOOD STABILIZERS

The medications in this group reduce or regulate mood swings of people with bipolar disorder (manic-depressive disorder). This group includes lithium (Eskalith, Lithonate, Lithobid, Lithane, and others), valproic acid (Depakene, Depakote), carbamazepine (Tegretol), and lamotrigine (Lamictal).

Lithium has been used to treat mood swings since the 1940s. Valproic acid and carbamazapine, both anti-convulsant medications originally used to treat epilepsy, have been widely used as mood stabilizers for two decades. Lamotrigine (Lamictal), another anti-convulsant medication, was approved by the FDA for maintenance treatment of bipolar disorder in 2003.

Lithium is considered the "gold standard" of bipolar disorder treatment. It is a naturally occurring substance. People taking lithium may experience nausea, diarrhea, abdominal cramps, muscle weakness and/or stiffness, hand tremor, headache, increased thirst, increased urination, weight gain, drowsiness, and fatigue. Most of these side effects are related to the level of medication in the blood. Blood levels should be checked, usually once or twice weekly at first, then monthly, and after six months to a year of stability, every two or three months. The dose needs to be adequate to control symptoms with the least amount of side effects. If any of these side effects suddenly gets worse, or if an unusual effect appears, the medication should be stopped and the physician called immediately. These changes could mean that the lithium blood level has entered the toxic range.

People taking valproic acid may experience nausea, vomiting, and indigestion. Valproic acid can also cause serious liver toxicity, although this is very rare. For this reason, people who take valproic acid must have periodic blood tests (approximately twice yearly after dosage has been adjusted).

Common side effects with lamotrigine (Lamictal) include dizziness, headache, blurred or double vision, lack of coordination, sleepiness, nausea, vomiting, insomnia, and rash. Although most people who develop rash have mild to moderate symptoms, some individuals may develop a serious or fatal skin reaction that requires hospitalization. Skin reactions are more likely if lamotrigine (Lamictal) is taken in combination with valproic acid (Depakote) or if the dose of lamotrigine (Lamictal) is too high. It is not possible to predict whether a mild rash will develop into a more serious reaction. If someone experiences a skin rash, hives, fever, swollen lymph glands, painful sores in the mouth or around the eyes, or swelling of lips or tongue, tell a doctor immediately. These symptoms may be the first signs of a serious or fatal reaction.

Several "atypical antipsychotic" medications are now being marketed for use in controlling mood swings. They were originally approved for cases when more traditional mood stabilizers were tried but found ineffective in relieving a person's symptoms. This group of medications is discussed at length earlier in this chapter. The FDA's approval of these medications for bipolar disorder does not mean that these medications are "better" than medications that have been used effectively for decades. Follow your doctor's advice about treatment.

STIMULANT MEDICATIONS

Stimulant medications are most often prescribed for attention deficit hyperactivity disorder (ADHD). The medications in this group include methylphenadate (Ritalin, Concerta, and Metadate), Adderall, dextroamphetamine (Dexedrine), and others.

These medications work by stimulating the central nervous system. This enhances certain focusing and filtering processes that occur in the brain. These functions tune out distractions, which helps people focus on what is important. When the tuning mechanism is not working correctly, people find it difficult to concentrate or control impulsive actions. Stimulant medication, in the right dosages, can calm hyperactivity and increase the ability to concentrate. Stimulant medications have been extensively studied. Information about their use in treatment of attention deficit disorder is widely available.

Most stimulant medications act quickly and stay in the body for relatively short periods. This makes it possible to time the dosage so the medication does not interfere with sleep. Extended-release versions of some stimulant medications are available. This allows people to take their medication once a day.

People taking these medications may experience loss of appetite, trouble sleeping, stomach pain, rapid heartbeat, possible slow growth pattern, dizziness, drowsiness, or changes in vision. People experiencing rapid heartbeat should contact the doctor immediately. Stimulant medications affect heart rate and increase blood pressure. People with heart conditions who take these medications have an increased risk of stroke, high blood pressure, heart palpitations, and arrhythmia. Stimulants can interact adversely with a variety of other medications. For example, people taking stimulant medication should avoid taking certain antihistamines and cold medications.

People with bipolar disorder can experience mood swings and mania when taking these medications. In rare cases, symptoms such as extreme irritability and even hallucinations can be attributable to the medication.

Strattera is a non-stimulant medication used for treating attention deficit disorder. The FDA has issued an advisory on Strattera, suggesting that parents and other caregivers watch closely for warning signs of suicide in children and teens taking this medicine.

Because stimulant medications can be abused and sold as street drugs, a written prescription may be required for each pharmacy refill.

MEDICATION NOTES

Many other medication side effects have not been included in the brief listings in this book. Every medication causes side effects. More information about medication is readily available in prescription information brochures, local libraries and on reference websites. When considering any medication, make sure to discuss the impact of the medication on overall health.

Adverse drug interactions are possible with any medication. Keep the doctor and pharmacy advised of all medications being taken, including over-the-counter medications.

Observe all warnings on the prescription bottle and the package insert. Many medications cause drowsiness or interfere with driving.

Avoid self-medicating with alcohol, over-the-counter medications and other supplements.

Many psychiatric medications increase vulnerability to heat-related complications such as heat stroke. It is critical that people taking psychiatric medications take appropriate steps to stay cool during hot weather.

Keep in touch with your doctor about how you are doing with the medication. Do not be afraid to tell your doctor about side effects or a desire to change medication. Call the doctor for advice on how or when to discontinue medication. Do not stop taking the medication just because you feel better. It is risky to adjust dosages or change psychiatric medication on your own.

NONCLINICAL RESOURCES

When people experience destructive thought patterns, they misinterpret what is happening, get stuck in negativity, or react physically to certain situations. Fortunately, people can confront these thought patterns and triggers, and gain substantial relief. This is an education process requiring guidance and practice. It is a major component of psychotherapy. Psychotherapy is a rich, meaningful experience, a guided, structured conversation within a professional relationship. Therapy helps people find new meaning in what they have experienced, and teaches new ways for people to move forward with their lives.

The resources that follow are written or supervised by clinicians, and designed around well-documented therapy techniques. They are intended for home or community use, or as supplements to psychiatric care.

Remember to check in with your medical team if you start using one of these resources. Do not use a book or community program as a substitute for appropriate medical advice.

Feeling Good: The New Mood Therapy by Dr. David Burns is cognitive behavioral therapy for depression in a book. The book's problem-solving and coping techniques can deliver rapid symptom improvement, and help with understanding, self-control, prevention of future symptoms, and personal growth. The book contains an overview of formal mood disorder treatment, and a guide to antidepressant drugs.

Stop Sabotaging: A 31-Day DBT Challenge to Change Your Life by Debbie Corso is based on Dialectical Behavior Therapy. Written by someone who has experienced Borderline Personality Disorder, the book aims to strengthen a person's ability to handle distress without losing control or acting destructively.

The Resilient Self: How Survivors of Troubled Families Rise Above Adversity by Steven J Wolin and Sybil Wolin is about resilience, the capacity to rebound from hardship or trauma. The authors' research shows that children of disturbed or incompetent parents learn to watch out for themselves, and grow strong in the process. The book focuses on a group of strengths and techniques that help resilient trauma survivors adapt and move forward. The authors invite readers to reframe their life experiences by focusing on achievements, not the trouble they have endured. This helps readers escape a victimized mindset, and sets the stage for a more satisfactory life.

Recovery International is a community group that uses cognitive therapy tools developed in the 1930s by Dr. Abraham Low. Group process is a key component of the Recovery International method. Like AA and other self-help groups, Recovery International meetings are organized and led by non-clinicians. Meetings are held regularly throughout the world. Participants review situations they have encountered, identify distorted thinking, and generate alternative strategies.

CHILD AND ADOLESCENT MENTAL HEALTH

Conversations about childhood mental illness easily deteriorate into partisan battles. Parents argue with other parents; doctors argue with other clinicians. Teachers sometimes lobby parents for medication solutions to fix a child's classroom behavior even if the law prohibits these demands. The popular literature can be even more confusing. Every position imaginable is reflected in the rhetoric of authors of books, magazine articles, TV talk shows, medical advertising, and internet sites. Unfortunately, despite the fact that the advice is so conflicting, everyone seems willing to dish out blame to parents as well as to children with disabilities.

PATTERNS OF DEVELOPMENT

The best approach to cutting through the rhetoric involves examining the normal development of children. This foundation helps differentiate normal variations among children from medical problems. Parents can also learn how making changes in the daily life of a child — simple changes like setting up social time, adding routines, adding physical activity, adjusting diet — can pay dividends in better child behavior. Understanding the wide range of normal and typical behavior helps parents and caregivers distinguish the sustained extremes of behavior that may require clinical intervention.

What behavior is normal for any particular child depends on the child's age, the child's stage of development, the child's culture, and many other factors. Every child's growth and development depends on complex biological processes driven by heredity, experience, family relationships, health, and culture. Child development is a process of growth, organization, and complexity. It is usually described as a process that moves sequentially, in stages. Each stage brings physical growth, new skills, and new patterns of behavior. Each stage is also part of a process that moves the child to maturity and adulthood.

As children experience life, they build their mental model of the world, and behave accordingly.

At each stage of development, children work through issues related to autonomy, the sense of being independent, and choosing one's own actions. This creates behavior that challenges parents and caregivers. A toddler's discovery of the word "no" is one step along the path to independence. A teenager's testing parental limits is another. These behaviors can be frustrating and distressing to parents, but they are normal, ordinary, and typical developmental milestones that are part of family life everywhere, in every culture.

Child development is organized into several areas called developmental domains. Developmental domains include physical growth and development; motor development; personal-social development; perceptual development; cognitive development; and language development. Each developmental domain depends on biological processes influenced by the circumstances and events in a child's life.

Issues and challenges in one area of development can affect any of the others. For example, a child's ability to speak depends on gaining control of the muscles of the mouth and tongue. Language skills also relate to social development. A child with autism may also have physical coordination issues.

Development requires practice and interaction with others. Without practice, one child's skills may lag behind another's. For example, a child without experience in group play may have trouble adapting to childcare or preschool. This relative inexperience shows up as frustrated, anxious, difficult behavior, but will usually work itself out over time.

Children grow and develop in predictable patterns, but they do so at their own pace. The range of what is normal for any particular child at any particular stage of development is very wide. For example, some children learn to walk at 11 months, while others walk at eighteen months. Every child has some area of development that lags behind the progress of some other children of similar age. This extremely common situation is termed a developmental delay. A delay can occur in any area of development, from speech to walking to social skills to cognitive skills. Most developmental delays resolve themselves in due course.

There is also a wide range of behavior that can be normal for children at any particular age. For example, some children may be more physically active or aggressive than others. Some children may be shy although their playmates are outgoing. This is all normal. We want and expect to see differences in children.

Although the overall pattern is somewhat predictable, child development hardly ever follows a straight path of progress. Children make progress, and then step back to behavior more typical of a younger child. For example, sick children act like younger children, needing more comfort or attention than usual.

Another way of looking at development is to see it as a process of children gaining normal functional control over their bodies and their lives. The reflex behaviors of infancy are replaced by voluntary control of movement and behavior.

BUILDING SUCCESS

What builds success? Current research indicates that the number one factor correlating with success in school is secure parental attachment in infancy. Responding promptly to infant distress helps children regulate their emotions, and promotes success throughout life. The second key factor is protection from traumatic experiences. Childhood trauma has lasting biological effects. It correlates with trouble in school, depression, and addiction problems later in life. Trauma has detrimental effects on children's ability to form relationships, as well as on executive function, the cognitive ability people use to solve problems when the way forward is not clear. A third factor prevents intellectual disability (formerly known as mental retardation). Abstaining from drinking alcohol while pregnant could eliminate most cases of intellectual disability in the United States.

Beyond these major preventative factors, the Search Institute has identified a list of 40 positive experiences and capacities that help children achieve success in life. The items on the list are called Developmental Assets. They are like money in the bank that children can rely on as they progress through life. These positive factors interact in a complex fashion to build resiliency and purpose. More of these assets means more likelihood of success. Having just a few assets correlates with more risky behavior and more trouble in life. Only a small portion of the assets relate directly to parents and immediate family. The rest are opportunities for others to pitch in. Among the items on the list are family support, positive adult role models, creative activities, youth programs, achievement motivation, safety, family boundaries, caring, reading for pleasure, homework, sense of purpose, conflict resolution skills, responsibility, and self-esteem. Learn more at www.search-institute.org.

FIRST SIGNS OF TROUBLE

Although children are routinely given screening tests to detect various physical problems, for example, hearing and vision tests, few screening tools measure childhood behavioral problems. These problems are typically detected by caregivers. When a child's behavior falls far outside what is normal for that child or for similar children of that age or developmental stage, caregivers may raise the issue with the parents and ask if the child might need to be referred for an evaluation. Reactions to requests like these will vary from parent to parent, but the news that one's child may have a serious problem is never completely welcome.

At this point, parents have an opportunity to try changing how the child is behaving. If you are in this position, consider keeping an informal diary or record of conduct that concerns you. This will be useful in the future when talking with doctors and educators. Be as specific as you can be with examples and dates. Do not neglect to keep track of your child's successes and good days! These are, in the long run, even more important than your child's "catalog of problems." Ask yourself, on the good days, "What helps our child succeed?"

IMPROVING BEHAVIOR

A variety of simple techniques can positively influence and calm childhood behavior. These techniques add structure to a child's day, reduce stress in the home environment, and encourage concentration, good daily health and nutrition. Trying them out can only help the situation.

Establish a fixed daily routine. Children benefit from consistency in day-to-day routines. Make sure there is a predictable pattern to your child's day. Follow a regular schedule from wake-up time to school/day care, to meal times and end-of-day rituals and bedtime. To the extent possible, follow the same routine every day.

Improve your family's diet. Adjust your meal habits to decrease intake of sugar and caffeine over the course of the day. Reduce or eliminate soda pop and juice, substituting water, especially late in the day. Increase the variety of foods you eat. Set and keep to a standard family mealtime.

Reject negativity. Force yourself to react resolutely positively with your child, even when the behavior is offensive, unacceptable, indefensible, hurtful, and wrong. The best approach is always to act calmly and controlled. Make sure the situation is kept safe, but do not react by escalating the situation. Yelling and name-calling make things worse. Remember that stress is poison to kids with mental health problems, so it makes sense to use discipline strategies that are calming instead of stressful. You want your child to learn control, and to see the benefits of remaining in control. This is not to say that you should not intervene. However, the response should be measured, and should always include an opportunity for the child to "process" the discipline. The basis for positive discipline techniques is a ritual of measured confrontation that interrupts the behavior and requires the child not only to "think about it" but also to express what was wrong, and apologize for it. There are many useful books on child discipline. Just remember that your point is to help your child learn control, and if there is a mental health problem, then learning control may be very difficult indeed.

Simplify the child's environment. Clutter and distraction can stress out children with mental health issues, and make it more difficult for them to think calmly or rest at the end of the day. Move TVs, computers, video game systems, cell phones and other "screens" out of the child's bedroom. Do not make this seem like punishment. Provide alternate places and times for the child to have access to these items. Tell the child that you simply want to provide a safe place that makes it easier for the child to feel restful and in control.

Lower the stress level at school. Tell teachers that you understand their concerns and are working to resolve the problem. If homework is a problem, carve out homework time each day and regulate it with a timer. It is better and easier to give all your attention directly to a child for one-half hour of homework time, than it is to force a child to wrestle with it for hours on end while you remain half-engaged yet vigilant. Besides, practically every child shares your desire to have the homework completed. Work on accomplishing more of it each day.

Recognize what your child achieves. Your child needs to experience your love, approval, and support.

All these techniques increase a child's sense of self-control, while reducing the burden of negative emotions and stress. These techniques are also safe, free, and harmless. They can be surprisingly effective.

It takes about 3 weeks to change a habit. Expect it to take that long before behavioral issues improve. Above all, do not be over-worried about keeping a perfect schedule, or the cleanest room, or the most rigorous diet, or even about becoming upset when things don't work out. You are simply trying to do as well as you can.

You are trying to "build up" a resilient, successful child, not "tear down" a problem.

CHILDHOOD BEHAVIORAL HEALTH EVALUATIONS

Behavioral health evaluations can involve any number of techniques.

Physical exams (including blood tests) begin the process, because every area of human development can affect behavior and emotions. Expect to encounter hearing and vision tests. Less frequently, children are referred for brain imaging or other medical scans or x-rays.

After the physical exam, families will encounter a variety of questionnaires. The questionnaires cover a family's history of inherited disorders, food allergies, the course of the pregnancy, pre-natal care, parental history of substance abuse, the parents' marital history, current living situation, ages when the child achieved various developmental milestones (turning over, walking, first words, first sentences), reading skill and school progress, nutritional habits, sleep patterns, and many other areas. Keep copies of everything you supply to the doctor. You may be able to "recycle" some of your work when you see a new clinician!

From time to time, a clinician may ask to observe a child during play or other activities at home, at school, at a daycare center or during play at a specially equipped office.

Many evaluations include "structured interviews." The doctor uses a list of set questions to guide discussions with the child or with caregivers. Each answer given leads to a new series of questions. Structured interviews help clinicians gather all the information that may be helpful for a diagnosis. These conversations will retrace information provided in the written questionnaires that have just been completed. Do not be offended when this happens. The idea is to get thorough information, and to discover material that did not make it to the paper questionnaires. Sometimes the structure of these interviews and the repetition helps parents and caregivers process the information in a way that improves understanding.

During the course of information gathering, the clinician will try to determine the nature of the problem. It helps to be specific, and to provide examples of the behavior that is the subject of the family's concern.

Do not expect to receive an answer or solution to your child's problem the first time you meet with a clinician. It takes time for the doctor to get to know your child and the situation, and to work out a diagnosis.

Most clinicians will encourage families to try one or more of the standard behavior-changing techniques before finalizing a diagnosis or suggesting a medical course of treatment.

Because there are no simple medical tests, and no universally successful, quick-acting, benign treatment strategies for childhood behavioral health issues, it is important to try what ordinarily works for the vast majority of children before resorting to other forms of treatment.

UNDERSTANDING YOUR CHILD'S DIAGNOSIS

A diagnosis will be based on factors listed in the catalog of mental health conditions used by clinicians: the Diagnostic and Statistical Manual or "DSM."

Most people expect a diagnosis to identify what is wrong with the child. Unfortunately, mental health diagnoses do not usually work that way. For the most part, the DSM diagnosis process is "functional" and not "organic." The diagnosis refers to aspects of how the person functions, not what is "organically wrong" with the person's brain.

Many disorders commonly identified in children reveal few clues about the nature of the biological process involved. For example, children may be given diagnoses such as an "adjustment disorder" (which means simply that the child cannot adapt to stressful events) or "conduct disorder" which is used to describe behavior that violates social norms. Neither label describes the biology of what is happening.

Other DSM diagnoses provide more clues to the organic nature of the person's ailment. Mood disorders, for example, are more associated with problems in the brain's limbic system. However, the brain is so complicated that pinpointing an area to "fix" is simply not a realistic proposition. Everything within the brain affects every other area in extremely subtle ways.

The DSM diagnosis is most useful for determining potential courses of treatment. This is because studies of the effectiveness of various treatments are correlated to specific DSM diagnostic listings. Studies show, for example, that lithium is very effective for people with the DSM diagnosis of bipolar disorder, but not as effective, or completely ineffective, as a treatment for many other DSM diagnoses.

What complicates the issue even more is that children's behavior can reflect features of more than one DSM diagnosis. Children may have more than one condition at a time, or partial symptoms of several disorders, some severe, others mild.

Your child might also be completely without mental illness, just active, frustrated, eccentric, or bored. We need to remember that every child is growing, and behavior always changes from time to time as the child progresses to adulthood. Many problems, even issues that are worth checking out, are simply not clinical disorders.

A CATALOG OF CHILDHOOD DISORDERS

Many issues relating to childhood mental illness are essentially unsettled. Common-sounding diagnoses may involve controversy and multiple schools of thought. Even when childhood mental health diagnoses have the same names as adult mental health diagnoses, adult symptoms differ from childhood symptoms. There is also debate over whether some childhood diagnostic labels even properly correlate with the same diagnostic label as applied to adults. Parents should also keep in mind that the DSM is revised periodically. Revisions in the DSM are widely debated even among clinicians. The following discussion focuses on some core areas where consensus exists.

Disorders of childhood and adolescence can affect a child's behavior and functioning at home or school. Every child's experience of mental and emotional health is unique. Some children experience features of one or more disorders that may be troublesome but may not rise to clinical levels of concern, while other children experience more of a match to the listings in a diagnostic manual, or might even have very severe levels of difficulty.

Many of the issues discussed in this section connect with difficult childhood experiences. Poor emotional attachment in infancy. Exposure to violence. Physical, emotional, or sexual abuse. Neglect. Loss of family members due to death, incarceration, or divorce. Any of these can lead to difficulty regulating emotions, difficulty forming emotional attachments, and cognitive problems, in particular problems with executive function, the ability to handle situations if there is no clear way forward.

Children benefit when family members commit to an appropriate role in treatment.

Mood disorders include bipolar disorder and childhood depression. Adults with depression are usually sad and withdrawn, but children may instead display aggressive or hostile behaviors. The "bipolar child" diagnosis is extremely controversial, in large part because antipsychotic medications are being heavily marketed (and some say overprescribed) to treat the condition. Yet some children do experience moods that shift from withdrawn and sad to aggressive, grandiose, violent and agitated, even shifting many times within a day. These children may indeed benefit from medication, treatment, and techniques designed to stabilize their moods. Parents should consider side effects and overall health when making medication decisions. Do not be afraid to research proposed treatments and discuss your concerns with your doctor. Do not rely solely on marketing materials when making medication decisions.

Anxiety disorders include school phobia, post-traumatic stress disorder, and avoidance disorder. The predominant feature in these disorders is exaggerated anxiety. In obsessive-compulsive disorder, the child feels the need to repeat an action over and over again.

Attention deficit hyperactivity disorder (ADD or ADHD) involves patterns of behavior that combine inattention, impulsivity, and sometimes hyperactivity. ADD symptoms overlap with those of several other childhood diagnoses. Some clinicians believe that ADD is a mild autistic spectrum disorder. Others may see the symptoms as childhood bipolar disorder. Many parents and clinicians believe that the condition is over-diagnosed, that normal active children are assigned this label primarily for the convenience of caregivers and school officials.

Thought disorders or psychoses involve thinking or mood that is extremely impaired and disconnected from external reality. The child experiences hallucinations or delusions.

Developmental disabilities. The terms "developmental disability" and "developmental disorder" refer to problems that arise during childhood and persist throughout life. Parents become aware of these problems when a developmental delay does not resolve itself, or when a child who has achieved a certain level of functioning takes a "step back," permanently losing skills the child once had.

Developmental disabilities can affect many key areas of a child's life, from self-care to social interactions to education. Children may face a combination of challenges in their lives, such as a developmental disorder combined with depression or another mental health problem. Each state maintains a system of supports and services for people with developmental disabilities and their families.

Intellectual disability (formerly termed mental retardation) is significantly sub-average intellectual functioning present from birth or early infancy, causing limitations in the ability to conduct normal activities of daily living. The ARC of the United States serves as an advocacy and support organization for people with intellectual disabilities and their families.

Autism spectrum disorders refer to a range of "social functioning" impairments that begin in early childhood and persist throughout adulthood. Autism affects communication and social interaction. The autism spectrum is very wide. Effects can range from very slight to highly disabling. Some children with autism develop repetitive behaviors, or have difficulty with creative or imaginative play. Most people with autism have difficulty reading body language or other nonverbal signals. Asperger's Syndrome is an autism variant characterized by highly developed language skills. Autism has historically been diagnosed around three to four years of age, but recently a variety of screening methods have allowed the condition to be diagnosed much earlier, as early as 12 to 14 months of age. Early diagnosis and remedial techniques can help increase a child's social functioning later in life. The techniques used to help with a child's social functioning resemble an intensified version of standard childcare.

Pervasive developmental disorder. Children with this diagnosis have problems in multiple areas of development. For example, a child may have difficulty processing information, may not speak, and may have poor motor skills and difficulty controlling movements. Doctors look for distortions, deviations, and delays in the development of social skills, motor skills, language, attention, perception, and reality testing. Physicians sometimes use this label as a "placeholder" until they can establish a firmer diagnosis.

Tourette syndrome is a persistent neurological disorder characterized by involuntary body movements and vocal outbursts (tics).

Learning disabilities are neurological disorders that make it difficult for a child to read printed words (dyslexia) or write using pen and pencil or a keyboard (dysgraphia), or do arithmetic (dyscalculia). Learning disorders are surprisingly common. A wide variety of technologies and techniques can help people address or compensate for the difficulties caused by these disorders.

Fetal Alcohol Syndrome and **Fetal Alcohol Effects** are neurological disorders caused by drinking during pregnancy. Drinking during pregnancy is the leading cause of intellectual disability in the U.S. Children of mothers who consume alcohol during pregnancy risk developing a variety of neurological issues, including difficulties with emotional attachment, lower intellectual functioning, and movement disorders.

SPECIAL EDUCATION

Both the Americans with Disabilities Act and Section 504 of the Rehabilitation Act prohibit discrimination against people with disabilities. These statutes require schools to make reasonable accommodations that permit children with disabilities to participate successfully in the educational program. These accommodations are relatively modest, for example, providing extra time with written tests or offering more frequent classroom breaks. Regulations implementing these statutes require schools to work out a written plan to accommodate the child's disability. These are sometimes referred to as "Section 504 Plans."

The Individuals with Disabilities in Education Act (IDEA) goes beyond prohibiting discrimination in education, including preschool education. IDEA entitles qualifying children with disabilities to the benefits of a "free and appropriate public education" in the "least restrictive environment." IDEA covers children with certain categories of disabilities.

- Autism
- Deafness
- Deaf-blindness
- Hearing impairment
- Mental retardation
- Multiple disabilities
- Orthopedic impairment
- Other health impairment
- Serious emotional disturbance
- Specific learning disability
- Speech or language impairment
- Traumatic brain injury

IDEA requires schools to identify and evaluate children to see if they have disabilities. Moreover, IDEA requires schools to provide educational supports, which can include tutors, special classes, speech and hearing services, and more. The IDEA requires schools to work with parents and students to develop an Individualized Education Plan (IEP) that outlines the nature of the disability, educational goals for the student, as well as the services the school will provide. This includes planning that helps the child transition out of high school to further education and a career.

Services required by the IDEA can be very expensive. It should not be surprising that parents, teachers, and school districts find themselves in conflict over what is appropriate for the individual child. Administrative hearings or appeals process, and even court intervention, are available to assist in resolving these disputes.

School districts can have good or horrible special education programs. Local disability advocates know their reputations. A variety of organizations and resources are available to assist parents as they advocate for their children in educational settings.

A child who graduates despite adversity has achieved a great victory.

TREATMENT AND MEDICATION FOR CHILDREN

Because children's brains are in "learning mode," interventions based on motivation, teaching, learning, and practice are usually successful with children. Children can learn to relax, focus, and attend to what is important. Social skills can also be practiced and learned. A child can be comforted, allowed additional physical activity, or offered a safe place in which to regain composure. These strategies help build resilience, and help the child to learn self-control. These strategies are necessary whether or not the child is taking medication to help treat the underlying medical condition. They build resiliency, which is essential for preventing problems in adult life. A good source of information about child resiliency is the Search Institute, which has developed techniques that build "developmental assets," or factors that improve a child's chances for a successful life.

Some children do need medication to stay safely in control of their emotions, or to be able to concentrate in school, or to make it possible to achieve their full potential in life. Committing to a course of medication is serious business. Parents should become informed and work consultatively with the medical team. People who care for children in foster care or substitute custody situations should be informed and accountable too.

Parents should realize that every medication causes side effects. Information about medication is available in local libraries and on reference websites. Take the time to research the specific medication that the medical team recommends. Do not rely solely on marketing materials when making medication decisions. When considering any medication, make sure to discuss the impact of the medication on the child's overall health.

Do not be afraid to discuss your concerns with your doctor. Each decision about medication should be carefully discussed and considered. Concerns about medication should not be dismissed lightly. Few psychiatric medications are FDA-approved for widespread childhood use. Nearly all have been developed and tested solely for adults. In addition, no psychotropic medication is entirely benign. Many medications carry warnings about long-term health effects. For example, antipsychotic medications, including "atypical" antipsychotics can cause a number of metabolic side effects (weight gain, diabetes, heart disease) which are very tough to manage. The long-term risks of many medications are simply unknown.

Consider asking the following questions. Why is a particular medication being suggested, when others are available? What are the side effects? What are the long-term effects on the child's growth and development? Has the medication been tested and approved by the FDA for use by children? What does the medication cost?

Take a moment to list the reasons for and against starting the proposed course of medication, and then make the best decision possible under the circumstances.

Monitor what happens as the family gains experience with the medication. Keep notes about how the child's life changes with the addition of medication. Maintain contact with the prescribing physician.

Parents should make decisions that they both can support, especially if a child has parents in separate households. Do not confuse your child or sabotage effective treatment.

PROGRESSING THROUGH ADULTHOOD

Young adults with disabilities have the same set of human needs, expectations, and capacities as everyone else. As young people learn to assume adult roles, they assert their autonomy, and establish their own identities. This process is awkward and troublesome, full of conflict, emotion, uncertainty, and drama. This transition to adulthood takes years.

The human development agenda cannot be ignored. People with disabilities make transitions too. Development may be at a different pace, and not every aspect of development may be in sync, but it unfolds nonetheless. Health issues complicate this process. As young people try on identities, they naturally reject the mantle of sickness and trouble, and everything that comes with it. Of course, this adds to conflict with parents, teachers, and clinicians, who rightly urge caution and attention to health.

The path through the transition years is part biology, part experience, part learning. Safe environments and positive relationships can help people build their adult identities, and flourish.

Safe environments satisfy essential biological needs, and tend to reduce stress and anxiety. Environments can be managed to support a person's individual needs. For example, many people with autism or mental health conditions are especially sensitive to distractions, randomness, and disorder. The author and scholar Temple Grandin, who has autism, turns off computer screen savers in rooms where she is working because the blinking and motion are visual danger triggers for her, and keep her at high alert. Grandin also avoids movies and television shows with cruel, violent content, because the images upset her and keep repeating in her head, even though she understands intellectually it is only theater and no one is being harmed.

People learn appropriate social roles through a process called modeling, mimicking the actions of others. Parents and adults in the community serve as role models, examples of how people succeed and live safely. Positive social models can even help with clinical issues. For example, young people who are prone to outbursts can learn to calm themselves by modeling the calm behavior of friends or relatives. Many young people benefit from art classes, soccer, group exercise, yoga, dancing, or martial arts. All of these deliver pro-social skills and use modeling as a key part of the program.

Environments should be safe, but not isolating. Isolation increases anxiety, reinforcing and perpetuating disability. Isolating young people stifles growth, prevents the development of adult friendships, and reduces opportunities for learning through modeling. Too much isolation creates risk, because friends and families cannot detect serious trouble. Concentrating people with disabilities into groups composed of individuals with similar problems reinforces self-stigma and an identity based on "differentness." Inevitably, people who spend most of their time in managed group situations see less of the larger world, and come to know fewer people in the general community.

LIVING THE SAFE MOVIE

People have always used stories, and even theater, to gain perspective and insight. These days it may sometimes help to think of life as a movie or video game that everyone is living out. This is just a shortcut, a technique that packages several complicated issues – issues like identity formation, goal setting, and risk-taking – together. What happens is real, and involves real people.

This becomes a simple way to plan a good future. If we can write our own movies, we can create our own best future. We can work things out as far as we can, play out our roles, and check in periodically, as matters progress. We can choose our timeframe and production team. We can choose the props we need, decide what motivates us. We can set our own goals.

Managing these elements generates context that helps us anticipate what might play out. After all, this is a theatrical technique, so why not rehearse. As we rehearse, we can ask more questions. How can we use what we are good at? What helps us make progress? What obstacles do we face? How can we stay safe? What endangers others? Rehearsing allows us to approach the toughest questions. What is our life's path? Can we find true love?

This technique promotes personal change. It may be time to change our movie, especially if we have had trouble in the past. We can work out how to make progress in a positive, safe world, and how to make peace with the people we love. We can see where situations are going, and reject options that are dangerous and risky. At any moment in life, we can change our movie, and become the best, kindest versions of ourselves.

THE SAFE ZONE SYSTEM

How do people learn to manage safety and exposure to the world? The Safe Zone System may help people who have difficulty with stressful or unfamiliar situations extend their range and stay safe. It boils safety down into a single question: Where can I be safe right now?

The Safe Zone System is a three-step process.

1. Classify places and situations into zones.

- Zone One is home base or "recovery space," where there is maximum safety.

- Zone Two is "routine space," familiar places like work or school.

- Zone Three is "adventure space," places with higher stress or stimulation.

2. Do a quick self-assessment. How am I doing right now?

3. Match capacity to space. Where can I be safe right now?

If you cannot be safe at the present zone level, move to the next lower zone or to recovery space. If you are having trouble in recovery space, contact someone for help.

The Safe Zone System must be customized for the individual person. It requires planning, rehearsal, coaching, and practice, but is simple enough to be written into IEPs and agency protocols.

This is a self-managed learning system. It is not a privilege or reward system. It is not a punishment system. Used properly, the Safe Zone System eliminates the need for restraints and time-out rooms.

ACCESSIBLE LANGUAGE, INTERPRETERS, AND ASSISTIVE DEVICES

Use accessible language to communicate with people who have cognitive disabilities. Accessible language is language free of jargon. Plain, nontechnical language, language that is concrete (for example, about physical objects or simple concepts). Eliminate metaphors when what you say will be taken literally. Be respectful. Do not use baby talk or teacher-voice. Speak at a normal volume.

If a person uses an interpreter, address the person, not the interpreter. The same rule applies to pictures and assistive devices. However interesting a picture, a device, or an interpreter might seem, it is the person in the conversation who requires your attention and respect.

Professional interpreters conform to an ethic that limits conversations with third parties in the presence of their client.

BEHAVIOR AND COMMUNICATION

For people with limited communication skills, unusual or difficult behavior can be a form of communication, a reaction to disappointment, discomfort, or disrespect. Fortunately, a person's capacities are never fixed. Difficult behavior decreases when people can access their strengths, satisfy their needs, and gain additional capacity.

DEPENDENCY AND SUGGESTIBILITY

People tend to lose capacity when they must depend on others.

Schools and social service systems tend to be authority driven, valuing compliance. People who spend time in these systems adapt to them, and learn to demonstrate compliance, at least superficially. People learn to say whatever authority figures want to hear.

People with intellectual disability often become dependent on others. They may become vulnerable to the power of suggestion, and can fall prey to the influence of protectors with dubious motives. Someone with a dominating influence can outmaneuver and exploit a person with intellectual disability.

People with intellectual disability can become conditioned to accept blame willingly, especially in situations where another person is involved.

People with intellectual disability often learn that smiles get approval, and that they are treated better when they appear to be happy. As a result, pleasant mannerisms may increase under pressure. The person may be trying to "get nicer" in order to navigate a stressful situation. People sometimes smile at inappropriate times, especially in the presence of someone in authority.

A HEALTHY LIFE, EVEN WITH LAYERS OF ISSUES

For people with co-occurring developmental disabilities and mental health disorders, environment and positive relationships still create the best path forward. Reduce noise and stress. Manage exposure to risky situations, but be willing to check things out.

Even if it takes longer to make progress, there is little to be gained from staying stuck. Find ways to contribute to family and community. Develop a positive story that takes care of the present, but still leaves room for progress and dreams.

People make progress when they focus on their strengths. The VIA Institute has a free online survey that can help start a conversation about anybody's "character strengths" (noncognitive skills like courage, love of learning, and determination). Learn more at www.viame.org.

ISSUES FOR OLDER ADULTS

Human development continues throughout life, even into older adulthood. People do not stop learning, adapting, or adjusting to new situations in life, even when they encounter health concerns. People retain or even build capacity if they stay active or keep using the capacities they have. However, if a person loses capacity because of injury or inactivity, it becomes increasingly difficult to regain it. Coping with an increase in dependency is always a challenge.

There is a directional pattern to gaining and losing capacity. In infancy, people typically gain control of their bodies from top to bottom, and from the center out. For example, a child gains control of his head and upper torso before he can walk or manipulate small objects. Older adults tend to lose capacity in the opposite direction. They may need assistance with mobility and fine motor control before needing help in other areas. At some point, it makes sense to adapt a person's home to reduce the likelihood of accidents and falls.

Although everyone tends to lose some capacity over time, loss of intellectual capacity is not normal, and neither is depression. These are medical issues. The earlier they are addressed, the greater the likelihood of recovery.

Dementia is a loss of intellectual capacity serious enough to interfere with a person's daily functioning. Dementia involves many types of brain function: memory, reasoning, thinking, even emotions. Dementia has many potential causes: Alzheimer's disease, stroke, advanced alcoholism, Huntington's disease or Parkinson's disease, even thyroid problems. A diagnostic work-up usually reveals the cause and determines the potential for treatment.

People adapt to the effects of memory loss. Some people ask others to supply information or help with reality testing. Others may be embarrassed, and try to conceal their memory loss. As memory declines, people may fill in gaps in memory with invented information. This is confabulation, a brain process that helps people maintain a sense of continuity or even identity. It is not the same as intentional lying. As people lose specific memories, they adapt to what they retain. This is what makes people with dementia appear to be living in the past. They are not retreating from today's circumstances. Instead, they are adapting to what they are experiencing. As far as they can determine, they are living in the chronological past.

Dementia can affect a person's personality. Many people with cognitive problems function better early in the day than they do at night. When the sun begins to go down, they may become more confused, agitated, and upset. This is called sundowning, a very common problem. Dementia also affects the capacity to regulate emotions. As people lose capacity, they focus more on non-verbal cues. They start modeling other people's emotions. They mimic other people's facial expressions and tone of voice, and internalize the apparent level of anxiety. People can also lose the ability to edit their expressions of emotion. Sometimes people appear much more upset than they really are.

People with dementia benefit from calm surroundings and good relationships with the people around them. Contact with elements of real life – children, friends, pets, gardens – is beneficial. Isolation is harmful, and loneliness is toxic. Busy commercial environments are usually too demanding. Address people with dementia with a soothing voice, relaxed posture, and serene facial expression. Do not be disrespectful or act as treat the person as a child. Do not try to force accurate information on someone whose thoughts are focused in another time. If the person is not interested in present-day "reality," address the person's emotional message. Solutions to sundowning vary from person to person, and sometimes from night to night for the same person. Some people need to release their anxiety through a brisk walk or other exercise. Others may need a hot bath, a back rub, or a glass of warm milk.

Even when they face significant challenges, people treasure their independence, and resent dependency. It is certainly appropriate to consider safety and risk, but, in order to preserve as much capacity for self-determination and autonomy as possible, always encourage people to do as much for themselves as they can.

PART TWO
ALLIES FOR RECOVERY

FINDING ALLIES

Support is essential to this fight. Isolation is a trap that makes people more vulnerable to the effects of the illness. Loneliness can lead to depression that has consequences for people with symptoms and caregivers alike. Do not reject the love, concern, and kindness of friends and family. Maintain your connections to the people you have always relied on for support.

Recruit new allies too.

You will certainly need a trusted guide for the process of recovery. Treatment systems are organized for this very purpose. Society is highly invested in medical and scientific expertise. We all understand that no system is perfect, and everyone has limits. What is your closest connection to the care that you may need?

Other allies are spread throughout our communities. Everyone has skills and talents, and people come together in every community to solve common problems. There are national advocacy groups with branches all across the country. Churches and faith-based groups also have a role. Who can you connect with in your city or your neighborhood?

Then there are our formal institutions. Libraries, parks, hospitals, businesses. All of these institutions have front doors you can walk through, and people to help you use their services.

If you type what you are looking for in an internet search box, and add the name of your town, you will discover many community groups and formal institutions that connect with important aspects of your life. No single place will have every answer.

Think about building a core team of allies, starting with the people in your life right now. Make a list of other people you can check in with on a more infrequent basis.

Who can you try to connect with right now?

FIGHTING FOR FAMILIES

When illness or hardship smacks into a family, a grief process can set in. We yearn for circumstances that will never return. We idealize what we have lost.

Sometimes we forget that every family hits tough times. No family is immune from stress or illness. No family handles adversity perfectly. We are becoming used to saying that families are becoming too fragile, but there is trouble within the strongest families. Even people who follow traditions and strive to lead model lives encounter trouble. There is power in the wedding vow. In sickness and in health.

Even though families are the natural form in which human beings organize to support and care for each other, accidents of history and many other factors have kept family life from much of the literature of mental illness recovery. Many early authors within the recovery movement were reacting to family members who forced them into abusive psychiatric hospitals. Even today, many authors who strongly oppose the medical model connect abuse they suffered in institutions with abuse they suffered in childhood.

The traditions of psychiatry also tend to separate individuals in treatment from allies within families. For example, we often fail to acknowledge limits to the usefulness of confidentiality. Professionals think it safer to withhold information even when they have discretion to share, making it more difficult to work through conflict. Power issues within institutions also take a toll. Poorly run treatment providers can manipulate information disclosure and other protocols to prevent concerned family members from assisting vulnerable patients.

Separating family members from people with symptoms is based more on faulty dogma and flawed tradition than on anything else. Even the best-intentioned people sometimes lose sight of stigma lurking below the surface of their programs.

We are not saying that people do not benefit from respite or from connecting with friends who are similarly situated. Those strategies do have power. Nevertheless, we firmly believe it is more important to work with the natural strengths of family life. Reconnecting with family members is an explicit goal of most treatment systems, yet people in recovery are often left to get there by themselves. Families that stay connected can focus on making progress.

Everyone in every family is entitled to make progress in their lives. It is natural to want to focus on the person who needs the most help, but over-focusing inevitably short-changes someone. Fortunately, family life is not a zero sum game. We can think more broadly about our problems. It pays to approach the issue more creatively.

Try asking the four recovery questions – but think about your whole family. What helps everyone make the most of their talents? What helps everyone reduce the areas where they are vulnerable? What helps everyone improve their capacity to handle stress? What helps everyone deal with the risk of something going wrong? This exercise literally keeps every family member on the same page.

Certainly there are situations where people's interests diverge, and families must consider difficult options. People who are dealing with very tough issues should obtain individualized advice from trusted professionals. If possible, talk with other people who have faced the same dilemma. The whole family benefits when everyone stays safe.

FOUR QUESTIONS AMONG FRIENDS

Friends everywhere help and support each other. Family, friends, and neighbors have relationships and social and cultural strengths that paid professionals cannot match. Often a friend or relative is the only person who can help.

Research shows that when people use the power of social relationships to work on problems together, they can solve the very toughest challenges.

Yet tough challenges are never easy, even when friends want the best for each other. Certainly it is normal for people to worry about what to do when a friend must face a difficult challenge or is experiencing difficult emotions. It is normal to become anxious about stepping in or stepping up.

We seldom talk about how to help or comfort the people we are closest to. Nobody teaches this. When someone is distraught, we might even feel ashamed we cannot help. We avoid pitching in. We look for rescue for ourselves, or we throw the ball to experts, even when it involves someone we love or a person we have known for years. We are capable of making all kinds of excuses to cover up our own uncertainty. We might say we do not want to make things worse.

As this human frailty builds up, people with problems become isolated. Our culture does not do a great job helping people talk about and work through their feelings. Everyone misses opportunities to pitch in and help.

Not to worry. Every culture on earth, and every religious tradition, supports helping people who are sick or in trouble. Everyone can learn simple ways to be supportive. This book has just enough to start.

Review the material that seems relevant, at a minimum the chapter on crisis and suicide, and identify someone you can call if you need backup. Beyond that, it is just a matter of resolve. Commit to helping your friend.

Here is one technique that screens for trouble and supports planning. It is a simple script, just four questions. This may seem artificial at first, but with five minutes of practice, you can follow the pattern using your own words. Remember, you want this to be supportive and voluntary. It is okay for this to feel awkward. Remember, you may be the only person in a position to offer support or head off trouble.

The goal of the script is to set a positive tone, support a person's engagement in a process of recovery, and screen for isolation and tunnel-vision thinking.

To get the best effect, find a quiet area. It is good to have others nearby, but out of earshot. Sit close enough to feel present with each other. Ask the questions one at a time, and wait for the person to answer.

Listen to the answers. Do not rush. People benefit when they say what they are dealing with, and benefit even more when they know they have been heard.

Ask these questions, in order.

1. What have you accomplished since the last time we met?

At a minimum, we both managed to show up for today's conversation.

2. What are you facing?

Let people identify their own challenges. Do not suggest answers. You can follow up by asking: "Why is that important?" Do not interrupt. Let the person finish.

3. Who are your allies?

Chances are that people already have someone helping them. If someone is all alone and has no allies, say that you will continue to check in with them and support them as much as you can.

4. What is your plan?

Let the person say what he plans to do. Do not jump in or interrupt. This is his plan, not yours. The minimum plan is to check in again at some future time.

Expect to experience some anxiety and unsettledness as you and your friend work through this script. That is normal. Life is a whole-body experience, and always connects with emotions.

Churches, schools, and community groups can incorporate this script into social gatherings or working sessions. You can use the questions as an icebreaker. Have people work in small groups of three or four.

These four questions apply to all sorts of challenges. There is no need to impose labels. They may help build a sense of community and support.

Do not make this script the whole point of your gathering. It is just there to help people stay safe and make progress.

However, if you have a strong reaction or fear about the person's safety, take action. You may be the only person able to help your friend. If there are any warning signs of suicide, ask about suicide directly. Say, "Are you thinking about killing yourself?" Stay with your friend if possible. Call your backup person. Take the next step for safety.

ACCESSING TREATMENT SYSTEMS

American healthcare in 2014 is in transition. The systems that deliver healthcare to most Americans are consolidating into large regional entities. State-financed systems are completing the transition to Medicaid funded systems. During 2013, in several states, people who depend on nonprofit providers that deliver community mental health services have found their services disrupted because their provider agencies encountered difficulties with audits. The Veteran's Administration has hired a large number of mental health professionals away from private sector practices. The Affordable Care Act and other parity legislation are equalizing reimbursement rates for mental health care. As events move forward, Americans will have more access to insurance, but there will also be more uncertainty about where to obtain treatment, because people who have new access will put additional pressure on the relatively small number of mental health providers in many U.S. communities. Many more people will soon have mental health coverage, but it takes time to build capacity to deliver mental health services. Expect this transition to last for several years.

In view of this system transition, people who need mental health treatment should double check their connection with their existing service system, and consider making backup plans. This is particularly important for people with chronic but moderate or controlled mental health issues. Systems under pressure tend to give priority to the most urgent cases. In 2013, several publicly funded systems reduced service for so-called low-priority clients. Emergency treatment remained available, but routine care suddenly became more difficult to arrange.

People who need mental health treatment should consider a multi-level relationship-building strategy. Work deliberately, but anticipate delays. It may take as long as six months to build relationships at every one of these levels.

- Nonclinical resources, such as support groups, advocacy groups, or pastoral counseling. Use these for support and for scouting out other local resources. Social support is not treatment, and is not a substitute for medical care. Social support is essential in its own right.

- Primary care systems. Establish a good relationship with a general practice physician or neighborhood clinic. Try to find a doctor who is willing to help manage access to mental health medication.

- Specialty outpatient resources. Find a counselor or therapist who will work with you and coordinate with your medical team on an as-needed basis. Case managers seldom provide psychotherapy. For medication management, find a psychiatrist who will collaborate with you and support the goals you set.

- Psychiatric emergency rooms. Make an informational visit to the local psychiatric emergency room. Become familiar with parking, with intake procedures, and with what is likely to happen if you must obtain services there.

The remainder of this chapter represents what "business as usual" looks like for people who require mental health care.

FIRST STEPS

Speedy action is important. Active symptoms lead to behavior with consequences.

Primary care physicians and hospital clinics can provide relatively prompt treatment at the onset of mental illness symptoms. If you do not have your own doctor, contact a neighborhood clinic for help, or a church-connected social service agency. Employee Assistance Plans (EAPs) also facilitate access to counseling or other treatment.

Most communities have an emergency room equipped to handle psychiatric emergencies. Local hospitals may be able to provide inpatient care to initiate treatment and stabilize the person.

It usually takes longer, potentially weeks, to reach an outpatient mental health specialist such as a psychiatrist, psychologist or social worker.

SPECIALIZED CARE

Private health insurers and managed care companies are the gatekeepers for private sector care. If you have private insurance, it is crucial to work with the company's care manager to ensure access to on-going services and payment of medical claims. Every health insurer has an appeals process to resolve disputes over treatment, claims, coverage, or eligibility.

Most health insurance plans require subscribers to choose from a roster of clinicians the insurance company has under contract. The care manager will usually send several names from the roster to people who wish to access service. Check out the providers on the list you receive with other people and professionals familiar with their approach to care. If there are no acceptable listed providers within your area, ask your plan's care manager to send another list, or permit you to select another provider of your choice at the "in-network" plan rate. Do not be surprised if you find that many providers are unwilling to accept new patients. You may need to rely on primary care doctors, emergency rooms, or community health centers for care while you work out access to a specialist.

Long-term inpatient hospitalization for mental illness is comparatively rare and expensive. Many people benefit from extended stays in residential treatment. People discharged from residential treatment before they are truly stabilized can deteriorate quickly. Their conduct becomes extremely disordered and disruptive. They frequently end up in jail.

COMMUNITY MENTAL HEALTH SYSTEM

The public sector mental health system is called the community mental health system. Usually a state department of mental health sets policy, and local county boards coordinate treatment. These local boards create plans for care that estimate community mental health treatment needs and specify the facilities and types of mental health services to be provided.

The state office is responsible for reviewing and approving these plans. Local boards then contract for services with local providers. Boards seldom provide mental health services themselves.

Community mental health services are funded through Medicaid, federal block grants, state budget appropriations, and, in some counties, through local property tax levies. Many local mental health boards also rely on product donations from pharmaceutical manufacturers for a significant portion of the medications they dispense. The availability of county levy dollars can result in much better access to care within the local community.

For information on receiving care through the public system, call the local mental health board. You will be referred to a local provider or to the community's "front door" for assessment and referral for care. Waiting times for services vary. Cases that are more urgent are handled first.

If there is a psychiatric emergency, go to your local hospital's emergency room.

CASE MANAGEMENT

Community mental health programs use a case management model, technically called "community support services," to coordinate care on an ongoing basis. People receiving mental health services through the public system (sometimes referred to as "consumers," a term originating in federal legislation) are assigned a case manager who coordinates treatment and provides a variety of other services. Case managers help with developing daily living skills. They assess needs and refer people for psychiatric evaluation and medication management, help with accessing public benefits, and assist with crisis management and stabilization. Case managers seldom provide individual or group psychotherapy.

People who need case management services have high levels of psychiatric impairment. Many public health systems only provide services to people who require this level of care.

Some areas have only one case management agency. Others have many. A good community support program will be recovery-oriented and focused on improving the lives of the people receiving services. Agencies are expected to involve family members, adopt a positive philosophy and work to connect people receiving services with social, leisure, and recreational activities in the community. On the other hand, cookie-cutter menus of standard services, indifferent staff members, and poor program management put vulnerable people at risk.

PEER SERVICES

Peer-to-peer support is very effective but underutilized. People with shared life experiences are powerful, effective allies. An easy way to connect with peer services is by calling a WARMLINE, a peer-run telephone listening line. You can find a list of toll-free national warmlines at www.warmline.org.

Trained Peer Specialists are sometimes paired with people leaving state hospitals to help with adjustment to life in the community. The Peer Bridger programs in New York have significantly reduced rehospitalizations.

Mutual support is the foundation of many therapeutic processes. For example, drug and alcohol mutual support groups build on the experience of people with shared experience of addiction. Shared experience and culture spurs personal growth and reinforces treatment.

Peer-delivered services are struggling to find a place in the developing mental healthcare ecosystem. The reluctance to fund peer delivered services is at least partially a remnant of mental illness stigma. Studies show that clinicians and administrators are as susceptible to stigma as anyone else is. Moreover, clinicians are experts who, as a group, prize their expertise and tend to devalue the work of nonclinicians. Western treatment traditions also insist on separating the private lives of therapist and client. A therapist is not permitted to be a client's friend, but peer services depend on friendship. This difference matters. Peer support is not watered-down therapy. It is explicitly social and relational. The barriers that protect therapy create problems in peer support work. In peer support, sharing is expected, because experiences and insights drawn from personal life matter the most. Another factor that keeps peer support from becoming more common relates to peer worker wage levels. In many treatment programs, clinicians earn high salaries, but certified peer specialists earn what cafeteria workers earn.

In a number of communities, people with mental illness run their own organizations that provide a range of services and activities. The clubhouse model combines mutual support, recreation, vocational training, personal advocacy and supported employment opportunities. Many community support agencies try to create pockets of peer-run programming within their organizational structures. The degree of true independence and self-determination within these "captive" programs varies greatly.

SUPPORT GROUPS

It is comforting to find people who relate to your situation. A support group helps defeat the feeling that you may be the only person in the world with these problems. It may be hard to find support from the people who are ordinarily the closest to you, especially if they lack knowledge, information, and perspective. Many people do not understand the difficulties of people with mental illness, or the challenges that family members face. This generates anxiety, social distance, and avoidance. People end up feeling lonely, hurt, and abandoned.

A support group may help you overcome problems and find hope. Support groups let people facing similar challenges help each other by sharing their concerns and frustrations, as well as practical ideas. People share the progress they are making, and discuss topics like housing, services, and treatment.

Many people drop into support groups for a few sessions, receive the answers and support they require, and then move on. Other people make lifelong friends. Many people attend support groups because they value opportunities to help others. They do not want other people to go through what they have experienced.

Support groups are informal, nonclinical and social. They are not the same as group therapy or 12-step groups. Meetings last an hour or so, and take place on a regular schedule.

ASSERTIVE COMMUNITY TREATMENT

Assertive Community Treatment (ACT) programs change the way communities deliver mental health services to people needing care. ACT was designed to serve people with mental illness who may otherwise be unable to care for their own needs. They are considered a "best practice" for people with severe mental illness who have the highest level of need. ACT clients may a high risk of recurring hospitalization, or have co-occurring substance abuse disorders or other health conditions, or may be experiencing homelessness.

ACT changes the way people with mental illness connect with the mental health system. Instead of seeing a case manager at an office, with occasional visits to a psychiatrist, care is handled by a team that includes the case manager, psychiatrist, nurse, and substance abuse professional if needed. The team acts assertively, bringing service to the person with mental illness, as well as educating family members about the illness and offering strategies to assist the person who needs care.

The word "assertive" does not mean "coercive." Assertive is merely the word used to signify that, when a person fails to appear for an appointment, the treatment team does not simply give up, sit in the office and wait for a crisis to bring the person back into care. Instead, team members work hard and consistently to connect with the person at home or in the community. Many studies have shown that ACT programs are both beneficial and cost-effective methods of engaging people with mental illness. They help sustain independence and progress in recovery.

DEPARTMENT OF VETERAN'S AFFAIRS (VA)

VA Medical Centers offers mental health and substance abuse treatment, as well as general medical care to military veterans. The VA has recently focused on effective treatment strategies for post-traumatic stress disorder. Some areas have better access to VA facilities than others do. For more information about VA Healthcare Benefits, contact local veteran's service organizations, such as AMVETS or Disabled American Veterans (DAV) or refer to the VA website www.va.gov.

COMMUNITY ORGANIZATIONS

Most communities have organizations that assist or advocate for people with mental illness and their families.

NATIONAL ORGANIZATIONS

Three national organizations stand out.

Mental Health America traces its origins to 1908. Clifford Beers started the group after writing a bestselling account of the degrading treatment and abuse he experienced while hospitalized after a suicide attempt. The organization's symbol is the 300-pound Mental Health Bell, which was cast from iron chains and shackles that had been used to restrain people with mental illness in asylums across the country. MHA promotes mental health and emphasizes recovery from mental illness. The organization has over 300 affiliates in 41 states and the District of Columbia.

NAMI (National Alliance on Mental Illness) was founded in 1979 by a small group of family members, and is now the largest organization focused on the needs of people with mental illness and their families. NAMI affiliates across the U.S. sponsor support groups and provide information services. Members appear on local television and radio shows, and speak publicly to educate others about mental illness. NAMI offers several community education programs. **Peer-to-Peer** is designed for people with serious mental illness. **Family-to-Family** is designed for family members and caregivers of people with mental illness. **NAMI Basics** focuses on issues faced by parents and caregivers of children and adolescents with mental illness. Each program promotes better understanding of mental illness and treatment, and helps participants through the kinds of difficulties they are likely to encounter. NAMI programs are team-taught, usually by volunteers, and delivered free. The education programs connect to ongoing support groups.

Recovery International is a community group that uses cognitive therapy tools developed in the 1930s by Dr. Abraham Low. Group process is a key component of the Recovery International method. Like AA and other self-help groups, Recovery International meetings are organized and led by non-clinicians. Meetings are held regularly throughout the world. Participants review situations they have encountered, identify distorted thinking, and generate alternative strategies.

WEBSITES

Many websites offer support and education. Remember that the Internet is a wild place. If you spend any amount of time looking for mental health resources on the Internet, you will certainly encounter conflict and controversy. The authors follow many blogs and news sites. We appreciate the diversity of opinion, and the courage of writers who are willing to share their struggle and offer advice. We view criticism of treatment systems, the medical model, pharmaceutical companies, and other major players in the world of mental health as a form of consumer protection, even when we do not agree with an author's point of view. We are amazed by the innovative thinking of people working in this field. We are often struck by the beauty of expression that we see.

Internet search engines have replaced phone books. For mental health treatment in your community, type "mental health treatment" or "mental health crisis" plus your town's name in any internet search box.

Network of Care, www.networkofcare.org links to many local resources as well as to social support.

If you have a child with a disability, try **Wrightslaw**, www.wrightslaw.com, which features coverage of special education topics.

ADDRESSING SHAME AND STIGMA

Allies are essential to reducing stigma and shame surrounding mental health issues. It is time to give up our natural tendency to hide or cover up our difficulties. Among the hallmarks of a diverse, just, and inclusive society are tolerance for difference, and support for everyone. Society changes as people live this out.

CONFRONTING SHAME

Once we get serious about our work with mental illness stigma and other tough social issues, we must eventually confront the topic of shame. This happens no matter how hard we have been steering away from it. Shame is the emotion that is left over, the disgusting ingredient on the cooking show menu.

People who design anti-stigma programs know that shame is not popular. We present graduate-level neuroscience seminars that never include a single mention of shame. We sometimes use stigma as a euphemism or code word to hide our discomfort with shame. This blockade on shame talk goes beyond our general reluctance to talk about our feelings (especially for men), but it is certainly connected. Nobody recommends using "what are you ashamed of?" as a pick-up line.

Fortunately, we have the work of Dr. Brené Brown to offer some clues about the shame component of mental illness and tough social problems. Brown uses a strict analytical process to talk about hard feelings, particularly shame. She does "qualitative" research – a process that involves collecting stories and looking for patterns. It lets her access a great deal of data based on people's real experience in the world – instead of merely tracking what happens in artificial, closed box situations.

Brown's work can help us distinguish between cognitive concepts and emotional experiences. For example, self-esteem is a thought about ourselves, a cognitive concept, while shame is an emotion, something we feel. Knowing how to work within this double dynamic becomes a kind of literacy.

Brown's key finding is that people experience shame as they encounter a "web of layered, conflicting, and competing social-community expectations that dictate who we should be, what we should be, and how we should be."

In other words, people get smacked with thoughts and emotions and cultural expectations all bundled together. Our emotions affect our thinking as we experience them in our gut. Our actions in response to shaming circumstances emerge from emotionally charged thought processes combined with our mental models and with what our culture expects us to be.

Dealing with feelings of fear, blame, and disconnection is difficult for everyone. You can imagine how tough this is for people with depression or another difficult illness, or for people who must depend on others for housing or material support.

Shame may be unwanted and disrespected as an emotion, but it is a common element in human experience. We cannot deny shame's existence. However, shame is an emotion with no constructive value. There is nothing good about it – and no "healthy" shame. Brown spent seven years testing the proposition that shame might be used to change people. She writes

It didn't take very long for me to reach the conclusion that there is nothing positive about shame. In any form, in any context and through any delivery system, shame is destructive. The idea that there are two types, healthy shame and toxic shame, did not bear out in any of my research.

The most effective response to shame is what Brown calls "shame resilience" – access to a process steeped in connection and empathy. The toxic opposites can involve "numbing out" – alcohol and drugs, isolation and despair. We perpetuate our own shame when we individualize ("I am the only one") or pathologize ("something is wrong with me") or reinforce ("I should be ashamed"). We perpetuate shame when we insulate ourselves (separating "us" and "them") or give ourselves permission to stereotype people.

Brown's research identified four key components of shame resiliency:

- The ability to recognize and understand shame triggers

- High levels of critical awareness

- The willingness to reach out to others

- The ability to speak shame.

Since shame comes bundled with our toughest social problems, and is always destructive, we should support shame resilience in the programs we design.

We can model shame resilience, designing messages that show people making connections and talking through problems.

We can emphasize commonality, not pathology, by showing how the experiences that make us feel the most alone are actually universal experiences.

We can scour our programming of common shame triggers. We might start by putting ordinary people, not professionals, at the center of our programs. Many people in Brown's research associated shame with education and helping professionals. According to Brown, the mere presence of a person with credentials in a room can have a shaming effect.

DISABILITY AND STIGMA

Shame connects with stigma, and with how our culture regards people with disabilities. Disability has three key aspects. One concerns visible or invisible differences between people compared to "normal." A second relates to a person's capacity to perform a range of tasks at home or work. The third aspect relates to the social regard for persons in such circumstances.

Everyone is subject to social processes that generate stereotypes, labels, and rules. People learn by modeling others. This generates social norms as well as stigmas. Every culture embodies explicit or implicit social rules about what to label as unsafe or shameful. As we learn how to live within our culture, we build our culture's rules about these stereotypes into our mental models of the world. Our mental models include rules about how to identify the stereotypes, rules about how to assign labels to people and situations that fit the stereotypes, and rules about how to treat people who have been tagged with the labels. Every human culture does this. It preserves tribal identity, and to a certain extent, it keeps people safe. Labels allow us to distinguish "them" from "us." We privilege "us," and penalize "them."

Stigma is one of the key factors leading to unequal treatment of groups in society. Stigma stereotypes facilitate social shaming. Labels have power. Because they develop and work through our social learning channel, they need not be rational. Shunning, shaming, exclusion, isolation, impoverishment, and incarceration are the default social penalties. Society rewards people who enforce social norms. People feel justified as they dish out social consequences.

Labels create socially reinforced blind spots, and hide what is valuable about people. Social policy often reinforces popular prejudices. For example, in the late 19th century, as the theory of evolution mixed with the era's crude racial stereotypes, researchers began to describe people with disabilities as regressions or throwbacks. This mode of thought, called Social Darwinism, set the stage for the eugenics movement and the Nazi Holocaust, and changed the mission of state institutions for people with mental illness and developmental disabilities. Asylums were originally promoted in the 1840s as moral reforms. However, by the early 20th century, Social Darwinism recast asylums as methods of social control. Asylums kept members of productive society safe and separated from those described as subnormal. People receiving care in these institutions suffered a kind of social death. Asylum inmates were rendered powerless. Clinicians dictated treatment, and "orderlies" controlled daily life. There is an unfortunate human tendency to dominate the powerless. People who confine and control stigmatized or disfavored populations easily turn abusive.

The disempowering effects of disability-connected stigma often lead to questions about what is best for people, and complicates decisions about care, and even about who deserves care. Stigma even denies people with disabilities the right to be regarded as experts about their own experiences. People with disabilities began asserting their claim for human rights following the struggles for racial and gender equality. The public remains uneasy with disability rights, especially the rights of people with mental health conditions. In the past, we isolated and confined people with mental illness in horrific institutions. Now we deny social resources to people with mental health conditions, and criminalize people who have difficulty managing their behavior when denied the resources necessary for their basic safety.

Mental illness stigma has several major patterns.

- Public stigma involves people who endorse the stigma and discriminate against people with mental illness.

- Self-stigma involves a person who internalizes negative stereotypes. Low self-esteem and low self-efficacy leads to self-blame, hopelessness, and helplessness.

- Label avoidance is stigma avoidance. People resist or defer treatment because they do not want to accept a shameful label.

- For caregivers and professionals there is another pattern, called "courtesy stigma." This is stigma by association. A person is devalued because they are close to people who have problems.

Fortunately, stigma disappears as people get to know each other. Social stereotypes are both created and destroyed through relationship-driven social learning.

The most effective anti-stigma efforts bring people together in ordinary social situations. This is called the social inclusion model. Anti-stigma campaigns that do not include social experiences are less effective.

We need to hang out with people to see past our blind spots. We soon begin to recognize the people that the labels are hiding.

ADVOCACY

Advocacy work protects people, corrects abuses, and helps people make progress.

Suffering, vulnerability, and stigma fuel the need for mental illness advocacy. People with mental illness are highly vulnerable to abuse, mistreatment, and ineffective care. The criminalization of people with mental illness remains unchecked. Public officials, hospital administrators, pharmaceutical companies, and health insurers have all demonstrated indifference to people with mental illness at one time or another. Even well intentioned experts may not know the right way to help a particular person.

SELF-ADVOCACY

Start with self-advocacy. Accept the care and concern of family and friends. Understand your rights. Set your own goals. Talk things over with people you trust.

Here are some suggestions for effective self-advocacy.

- Do not be afraid or ashamed to acknowledge that you are engaged in recovery from a bout of mental illness. This is the first step in eliminating stigma.

- Try to keep a record of everything you do. List names, addresses, phone numbers, email addresses, dates of crisis events, admission to hospitals, medication administered, and dates of discharge. Make notes of conversations and conferences. Make copies of everything you mail. Keep all notices and letters, and copies of all your emails.

- If you encounter abuse on the part of a clinician or treatment agency, refer to the section on complaints and grievances. People are entitled to adequate treatment. You should not be satisfied with less.

- Write letters of appreciation when warranted. When necessary, write letters of criticism. Send these to the hospital or agency director, with copies to anyone else who may be involved. If services are very inadequate, send copies to your legislator or other state officials.

- Do not accept a vague answer or statement that seems confusing. Pursue a clarification if you feel you do not understand.

Above all, be assertive yet measured in your approach to self-advocacy. You are entitled to information, respect, and courtesy. Treatment agencies say they want to provide person-centered care. Public agencies strive to show they are accountable, good stewards of public resources. You are not asking for favors.

INFORMAL PERSONAL ADVOCACY

Informal personal advocacy starts with kindness, loyalty, and the willingness to learn. If you are collaborating with a family member, expect old history and disappointments to creep up as you struggle with today's issues. Try to focus on shared goals.

The author Wendy Lustbader writes eloquently about what she calls the dance of guilt and resentment. It is painful to become dependent, painful to see another person becoming dependent, and frustrating to realize that you can never adequately fill the hole created by another person's need.

FORMAL ADVOCACY

Formal advocates are authorized to speak or act on behalf of another person. Loyalty is paramount. Expertise helps too. People do benefit when an institution must respond or account to a formal advocate. There is a wide range of formal advocacy roles, starting with having written authorization to access information. Roles that are more powerful include assisting with a claim for benefits, or having a voice in treatment decisions if a person becomes incapacitated.

When speaking to clinicians, be polite and keep conversations to the point. Do not try to intimidate the members of the treatment team and do not allow yourself to be intimidated. Clinicians have a strong interest in their client's health. They try to respond to the concerns of family members. Treatment teams nearly always support family-connected strategies that help the person receiving treatment.

People in treatment who want other people to help them work with the treatment team will need to provide written permission to review medical records and speak with clinicians about treatment matters. No one can provide effective assistance without written permission from the person receiving treatment.

If you are assisting another person, keep the person informed about everything you plan to do, especially if you are that person's guardian. The person might disapprove of what you plan to do about treatment, placement, finances, or medication, or may wish to have the situation handled differently.

PUBLIC ADVOCACY

Public advocacy means communicating about the needs of people with mental illness through public speech or writing. Personal testimony is a powerful tool, as essential as statistics, brain scans, and charts. Education is another public advocacy strategy. Every time you write a letter to the editor or send an article, you are doing public advocacy.

LEGISLATIVE ADVOCACY

Legislative advocacy is easier than you might think. Legislators try to be responsive to their constituents. Internet tools now make public officials more accessible than ever before.

Be informed. Read newsletters and legislative/advocacy alerts carefully. Know both sides of the issues. Know when the bill is in committee, when the hearings will be held, and who the co-sponsors are.

Start early. Pay attention to issues and proposals early in the process and you will have a better chance of affecting the outcome.

Be concise. The more simply and clearly you explain your position, the better chance you have of getting people to listen and respond.

Be specific. Know exactly what you want your legislator to do. Do you want the legislator to draft legislation? Propose an amendment? Vote for the bill?

Be honest. Do not exaggerate to make a point or answer a question if you are not sure of the facts. Every issue has at least two sides. Be honest about admitting the pros and cons of your issue.

Give personal examples. This puts the issues in memorable, human terms. Saying that you or a family member went without dinner for a week because there was not enough money to buy food is much more powerful than giving statistics that show that SSI recipients are living below the poverty level.

Practice. Try explaining your position to friends and family before you meet with a legislator or testify before a committee.

Communicate with your legislative network contact. Tell them what your legislator said, so that network can follow-up appropriately.

Be courteous, but firm and confident.

Do not make threats. Telling legislators that they have to do what you want or you will not vote for them only turns people off.

Do not argue with your legislator. If it is clear that the person will not support your position, just give the facts and ask him or her to consider your viewpoint. You want to keep the lines of communication open for discussing future issues.

Do not give up.

COMPLAINTS AND GRIEVANCES

Both people in treatment and family members can initiate grievances about community mental health services. Written permission will eventually be needed for a representative or family member to access treatment records.

Begin by discussing the problem with the agency case manager or therapist. If this does not resolve the issue, contact a supervisor or the director of the mental health agency or facility.

Information about an agency's grievance procedure is usually distributed at intake and posted on facility bulletin boards. Follow the steps in the procedure. If your complaint is not resolved, the way you want it to be, you can usually appeal to a higher agency official, or request mediation, or file a further grievance. Every community mental health board has a client rights officer who can assist in resolving grievances. You may also be able to get help from state and federal regulatory agencies. Be especially aware of time limits.

If the problem seems to be a violation of professional ethics or law, contact the ethics committee of the relevant professional organization. Treatment agencies are also monitored by national accrediting organizations that may offer avenues for engaging agency officials and solving the problem.

For help with grievances, contact your state's disability advocacy group or public advocacy groups like Legal Aid. Type "disability advocate" and the name of your state in an internet search box for more information about services that may be available to you.

PART THREE
FINDING RESOURCES

PAYING FOR MENTAL HEALTH SERVICES

Even with the rollout of the Affordable Care Act, and the expansion of Medicaid in many states, many people with mental illness will continue to have difficulty obtaining adequate levels of healthcare coverage. It has been lawful for health insurance companies to systematically divert people with mental illness from their benefit rolls by capping services, excluding diagnostic categories from coverage, and underpaying for services to the point where private therapists refuse to contract with managed care groups. Recent legislation has alleviated some of this, but has not solved the problem. During the next few years, more people will have insurance coverage, but the system will still have about the same capacity to deliver mental health appointments.

HEALTH INSURANCE COVERAGE

People with mental illness should take advantage of opportunities to enroll for coverage under the national or state health insurance exchanges. Coverage varies from plan to plan. Employer plans are transitioning to the point where they provide adequate coverage for mental health care.

People with good insurance coverage should work hard to retain it. Private insurance is a key element in gaining prompt access to treatment. Because it takes weeks for nearly any mental health treatment to work, the typical six-week delay before being seen by a public system therapist results in work and family disruption that lasts a minimum of three months. As the Affordable Care Act begins to increase reimbursements for mental health care, local private sector therapists and clinics will begin to experience increased demand for appointments. Until the healthcare system stabilizes, access to specialized care will continue to be difficult, even in communities that are comparatively better-served.

People who become aware of the potential need for high-expense residential treatment should contact a lawyer for advice about this as soon as possible. Health insurance plans limit payment for lengthy episodes of inpatient hospital or residential healthcare. If you encounter a need for this level of care, you must prepare for the possibility that you will be forced to liquidate personal or family assets before seeking help from publicly financed payment sources such as Medicaid.

MEDICAID

Medicaid is the largest funder of mental health services in the United States. Although there are minimum coverage and benefit levels, the administration of Medicaid and the services covered vary substantially depending on the particular state plan. Medicaid is a health insurance program for people with low income and limited assets. Although the majority of people enrolled in Medicaid are young families and children without disabilities, the majority of Medicaid expenditures pay for services to people who are aged, blind, or disabled.

People who receive SSI are automatically eligible for Medicaid. Many disabled people who do not receive SSI, but who have low incomes, may still be eligible for Medicaid. One way is through spend-down, which means using a portion of income to pay for medical expenses. After that point, the person becomes eligible for Medicaid coverage for the remainder of the month.

The local county welfare office usually handles applications for Medicaid.

Medicaid benefits vary substantially from state to state. Only 45 percent of poor Americans are covered by Medicaid. The federal government requires that each state cover certain specific populations, but many states do not choose to cover every beneficiary category the program allows. There is a limited menu of mandatory covered services as well, such as hospital and nursing home care. Other than that, each state can choose the medical services to be covered from a list of so-called "optional services." States can even customize their Medicaid programs by asking the federal government to waive otherwise mandatory program provisions.

Many states use Medicaid to pay for a wide range of optional services, including community alcohol and other drug addiction treatment services, community mental health services, and prescription drugs. Other states choose to cover many fewer services. People who need services that are not included in the state

Medicaid plan must find a way to obtain them on the open market or through charity groups – or simply go without care. Many Americans have poorer health because they cannot afford needed (let alone optimal) medical care.

The advent of managed care makes Medicaid even more difficult to navigate for many individuals. Managed care organizations require approvals for various types of care and limit access to expensive medication. Because newer psychiatric medication is so expensive, many managed care plans restrict availability of these drugs. Because people with mental illness have less capacity to deal with the stress of navigating complicated systems, their health is put at substantial risk by these restrictions. Medicaid is funded jointly by the federal government and state governments. The amount of funding each state receives depends on the actual amount spent for Medicaid services. Each state has to provide a certain amount of "matching funds" in order to receive the federal reimbursement.

Medicaid spending is one of the largest categories of spending in state budgets. Increases in Medicaid program costs can seriously affect the fiscal condition of the state. When state budgets are cut, states reduce the number of optional Medicaid services they pay for, and restrict eligibility to people with extremely low income.

Medicaid is intended for the nation's poorest citizens. It provides care not covered by other types of insurance, particularly long-term care in nursing homes. However, Medicaid is intended to be a payer of last resort. People are expected to use nearly all their income and their other assets before receiving benefits from Medicaid. Program rules outlaw asset transfers that create eligibility for coverage. People who know they may face a need for long-term care will benefit from consulting with a so-called elder law attorney as soon as possible, in order to preserve assets in a fashion that meets legal requirements and protects other family members. Spouses of individuals who need nursing home care are particularly vulnerable to asset look-back provisions.

MEDICARE

Medicare is the basic federal health insurance program for people over 65 and for many people with disabilities. People age 65 and older who qualify for Social Security retirement benefits are automatically eligible for Medicare. After 24 months, people who receive Social Security Disability Insurance Benefits qualify for Medicare.

Medicare Part A covers hospital care and some follow-up services, skilled nursing facility care, and hospice care. For Medicare Part A, which pays for inpatient hospital, skilled nursing facility, and some home health care, the deductible paid by the beneficiary is $1184 in 2014. The Part A deductible is the beneficiary's only cost for up to 60 days of Medicare-covered inpatient hospital care. However, for extended Medicare-covered hospital stays, beneficiaries must pay an additional $296 per day for days 61 through 90 in 2014, and $608 per day for hospital stays beyond the 90th day in a benefit period. For beneficiaries in skilled nursing facilities, the daily co-insurance for days 21 through 100 is $148 in 2014.

Most Medicare beneficiaries do not pay a premium for Part A services since they have 40 quarters of Medicare-covered employment. Other seniors and certain people under age 65 with disabilities may obtain Part A coverage by paying a monthly premium set according to a formula in the Medicare statute.

Medicare Part B covers doctors' visits, lab tests, outpatient services, and medical supplies. Part B is optional insurance, and must be paid for by the individual. For most individuals, the 2014 monthly cost of Part B is $104.90.

Medicare does not pay for dental care, eye care, routine check-ups, or medications. Therefore, many recipients also carry private insurance.

Medicare historically paid a smaller percentage of mental-health related costs than it pays for other types of care. The Affordable Care Act is equalizing reimbursement rates. Medicare Part B typically pays 80 percent of the amount of the fee that it approves. Payments start after the beneficiary pays an annual deductible ($147 in 2014).

Medicare Part C is known as Medicare Advantage. Medicare Advantage Plans are offered by private companies that contract with Medicare to provide beneficiaries with both Part A and Part B benefits. Medicare advantage plans vary substantially, and include health maintenance organizations, preferred provider organizations, private fee-for-service plans, special needs plans, and Medicare medical savings account plans. For people enrolled in Medicare Advantage plans, services are covered through the plan and are not paid for under original Medicare. Most Medicare Advantage plans offer prescription drug coverage. Because the plans are so diverse, it is important to choose one with the proper mix of providers and benefits.

Medicare Part D provides coverage of prescription drug expenses. Eligible beneficiaries select from a variety of vendor plans. The system is complicated, and sometimes difficult to navigate. People with mental illness have experienced great difficulty accessing psychiatric medications under these plans. According to the Medicare Rights Center, despite instruction from the Centers for Medicare and Medicaid Services (CMS) to Medicare Part D plan providers to cover substantially all mental health drugs, many plans either have failed to provide coverage or have instituted utilization management techniques that restrict consumer access to antidepressant and antipsychotic medications. Nearly one out of four common antidepressant and antipsychotic medications are subject to utilization management or are absent from Part D plan formularies. Many plans apply utilization management differently depending on whether the drug is generic or brand name. Higher-priced drugs often have higher rates of utilization management. People with mental illness find it more difficult than others to navigate the bureaucratic process that is required to obtain coverage for restricted drugs. The frustrations and stress can lead patients with mental illness to abandon their medication regimens and decompensate.

Medicare and Medicaid programs interact in complex ways. Special programs pay some or all of Medicaid beneficiaries' Medicare premiums and coinsurance costs. So-called dual eligible have been transitioning to maximize use of Medicare to fund their healthcare costs.

The best sources of information about Medicare coverage and benefits are advocacy groups such as the AARP and the Medicare Rights Center.

HOUSING

Everyone needs safe, affordable, and decent housing. People with mental illness should have the same housing options as everyone else. They should be able to decide where and with whom they live.

Economic factors are the most important determinants of housing quality. Effective, timely treatment and family support work together to preserve the economic capacity of people with mental illness. Maintaining this capacity is an urgent concern.

If treatment and family support are not enough, homelessness prevention programs matched with case management can help people with mental illness retain their housing or locate decent subsidized housing. Local community mental health agencies have a designated housing coordinator who can provide information about where to begin the search for appropriate housing.

Unfortunately, many people with mental illness reside in substandard housing. Finding good housing for a person with mental illness is challenging. The key factor is poverty. For people with severe mental illness, good housing usually means housing that is subsidized in some way. People with severe mental illness are very likely to be unemployed or underemployed. Even if they become entitled to disability benefits, their income is rarely sufficient to provide good housing. The federal SSI benefit for an individual does not provide enough income for a market-rate apartment anywhere in the United States.

Home ownership is an important option. People with disabilities may be able to retain their homes with some level of support from family or from local housing assistance programs. People can sometimes use their property or reverse mortgage programs to generate an income stream for self-support. Make sure to obtain qualified financial and legal advice when considering these options.

Private apartments require stable sources of income. Some property owners participate in voucher-based housing programs. A voucher is a government check to the property owner for a portion of the tenant's rent. The tenant pays the rest of the rent. Most housing for people with mental illness is voucher-based. Special federal and state programs, such as the U.S. Department of Housing and Urban Development's Section 8 program, cover the cost of the vouchers. Housing coordinators in local community mental health agencies can help connect you to the agency that manages housing vouchers in your area.

Public housing projects are apartment complexes or developments in which all units are owned and operated by a public housing authority. Some private developers use government housing program funds to develop apartments, and agree to make apartments available to subsidized public housing clients in return. Tenants pay rent based on an income scale set by federal regulations. These projects are seldom devoted solely to people with disabilities. In general, no supportive services are associated with the housing. A person living in public housing will continue to receive services from the community mental health system.

HOMELESS ASSISTANCE PROGRAMS

Many homeless people have mental illness and/or substance abuse problems that contribute to the person's lack of stable housing. Housing and social service agencies work together on a county or regional level, using federal and other funds to deploy both case management services and a range of housing types, from one-night shelters to apartments to single-family homes. The menu of housing choices and the way programs are administered varies considerably from location to location.

Shelter programs provide temporary or emergency housing for a brief period of time (a day or a week, rarely as long as a month). The availability of shelter programs varies widely across the United States. Many shelters use a night-only model. Shelter residents must leave every morning with all of their possessions. Some programs can accommodate young children. Families that include older male children have the most difficulty finding emergency shelter.

Transitional housing programs move homeless people into permanent housing within a relatively brief time, typically measured in months. The facility assists in finding income, resources and supports that will make it possible to live in permanent housing. This category includes many residential treatment facilities and halfway houses serving people recovering from substance abuse or recently released prisoners.

Housing First is a program model that places clients in permanent housing, and then adds services and supports. Housing is a major stabilizing factor in a person's life.

TREATMENT SETTINGS

Residential treatment facilities restrict a person's freedom in addition to providing costly services. They are appropriate placements only so long as the person needs the level of care that is provided. People who receive residential care for long periods of time stop practicing the daily tasks of living on their own. They risk becoming dependent on the facility's support and routine, and may develop an institutionalized, dependent mindset that makes transition to independent living difficult. The Americans with Disabilities Act and a series of judicial rulings require states to deliver treatment in the least restrictive setting. Community settings are always preferred.

The institutions described in this section are frequently encountered within mental illness treatment systems. People with developmental disabilities, people involved in the criminal justice system, and people receiving services through the alcohol and drug addiction services system may receive treatment in other types of facilities.

State hospitals provide care to people found to be a danger to self or others, or with substantial mental illness issues and criminal justice system involvement. Placement in a state hospital is seldom voluntary.

Very few private hospitals provide long-term residential mental health services.

Hospital acute care units are secure facilities within community hospitals used primarily for mental health emergencies. Stays in these units are generally very short. Treatment is usually covered by contracts with private insurance carriers, Medicare, Medicaid, or local mental health boards. Community hospitals also provide a great deal of uncompensated care to people with mental illness.

NURSING HOMES

Nursing homes are designed to provide continuing medical care to people with severe medical conditions. Nursing home care is very expensive, and constitutes one of the largest components of Medicaid spending. People with mental illness and other medical conditions sometimes require nursing home care. However, because of the scarcity of subsidized community housing, there is pressure to use nursing homes for people with mental illness more frequently than necessary.

Many advocates fear that nursing homes are becoming the modern equivalent of the back wards of the large state institutions of the past. In 2004 (the most recent data currently available) there were nearly 1 million nursing home residents in the US with a primary mental illness diagnosis. Only ten percent of these residents had senile dementia or an organic brain disorder. An additional 1.4 million nursing home residents had Alzheimer's disease, Parkinson's disease or other neurological disorders as their primary diagnosis.

Some nursing homes are known to discharge difficult clients and retain easier clients that do not need nursing home levels of care. Many states review all admissions of people with mental illness to nursing homes.

GROUP HOMES (ADULT CARE FACILITIES)

When three or more unrelated individuals share a house or other facility this is termed a "group home" or adult care facility (ACF). ACFs are required to provide a certain degree of private space for residents, together with shared facilities for meals and socializing. Each ACF is required to provide some minimal level of staffing and supervision.

Each state has a way to regulate care and safety of ACFs. Sometimes these homes are just part of a catchall category of facilities not regulated by other entities. Nursing homes, mental health residential treatment facilities, drug and alcohol addiction programs, and halfway houses have much stricter regulation than ACFs.

The quality of ACFs varies widely. Some ACF operators take great pride in their work and provide good service and a high quality of life for their residents. Other ACF operators seem to be driven by greed, offering only squalor and dehumanizing conditions. Inspections rarely result in fines against unscrupulous operators.

Rules that protect vulnerable people from exploitation vary in effectiveness from state to state. Continuity of care can be a problem, especially when one county places an individual in an out-of-county ACF. Mental health system workers sometimes drop the ball when arranging for care during and after transition. In these cases, people needing care can find themselves without access to treatment, case management, or medication.

When a person is referred to an ACF by a mental health agency, the agency should develop a written, individualized mental health plan to help make sure the placement is safe and supportive. The plan should address medication and possible adverse side effects, personal care services or other assistance the person needs, and the entity that is to provide these services. The plan should ensure that the person remains connected to services and to the person's family. The plan should also address what will happen in the event of emergencies, including advance directives such as living wills or powers of attorney for health care. The plan should be updated at least once a year.

If you are helping a friend or family member who is being referred to an ACF, you can become involved in the process and advocate for your friend or relative during the preparation of the plan for care. Know who the responsible case management agency is and how to reach them in case of emergencies.

People entering ACFs should have a medical evaluation to make sure the level of care provided by the facility is matched to the level of service the person requires. Follow-up exams should take place every year. People in ACFs need to be able to self-administer prescribed medication. The resident and the ACF need to know about special dietary requirements and other health concerns, including tuberculosis and other infectious disease exposure.

ACFs receive rent payments from residents, and sometimes money from supplemental state funding programs. The amount of pocket money remaining available to a resident varies widely within ACFs based on state rules. Some residents may be able to keep nearly all of their income, while others struggle to keep small amounts of cash for cigarettes and snacks. Friends and relatives can help ensure that ACF residents retain access to personal resources.

The best ACFs maintain close ties to with community mental health treatment agencies that provide case management and other services for residents. Good case managers visit regularly, inspect living quarters, and speak with their clients privately on a regular basis.

Be sensitive to issues of abuse and neglect. People who require group home placement are vulnerable to abuse and exploitation. Resident-to-resident abuse can be a very serious problem. Sometimes residents loan others cigarettes or snacks and then take the resident's checks at the beginning of each month, or steal property. Sexual abuse sometimes occurs. There may be no planned activities. Some case managers seldom visit.

State law governs the rights of people living in ACFs. There are some common elements. Before admission, the resident should sign, and the facility should explain, the terms of a resident agreement that sets out all charges that apply. The resident should have their own copy of the signed agreement. Arrangements should be made concerning how the resident will continue to connect with mental health and medical services. The ACF should explain its resident's rights policies and procedures, and provide written copies of rules and procedures. In addition to day-to-day rules for meals, sleeping arrangements and fire safety, the written material should include the process the facility uses when making referrals for mental health and medical evaluations.

Some states have explicit lists of rights of ACF residents. Ohio's list includes the following.

- The right to a safe, healthy, clean, and decent living environment.

- The right to be treated at all times with courtesy and respect, and with full recognition of — personal dignity and individuality.

- The right to practice a religion of his or her choice or to abstain from the practice of religion.

- The right to manage personal financial affairs.

- The right to retain and use personal clothing.

- The right to ownership and reasonable use of personal property so as to maintain personal dignity and individuality.

- The right to participate in activities within the facility and to use the common areas of the facility.

- The right to engage in or refrain from engaging in activities of his or her own choosing within reason.

- The right to private and unrestricted communications, including the right to receive, send, and mail sealed, unopened correspondence, the right to reasonable access to a telephone for private communications, and the right to private visits at any reasonable hour.

- The right to initiate and maintain contact with the community, including the right to participate in the activities of community groups at his or her initiative or at the initiative of community groups.

- The right to state grievances to the owner or the manager of the facility, to any governmental agency, or to any other person without reprisal.

- Prior to becoming a resident, the right to visit the facility alone or with his or her sponsor.

- The right to retain the services of any health or social services practitioner at his or her own expense.

- The right to refuse medical treatment or services, or if the resident has been adjudicated incompetent and has not been restored to legal capacity, the right to have his legal guardian make decisions about medical treatment and services for him or her.

- The right to be free from abuse, neglect, or exploitation.

- The right to be free from physical restraints.

- The right not to be deprived of any legal rights solely by reason of residence in an adult care facility.

- The right to examine records maintained by the adult care facility concerning him or her, upon request.

- The right to confidential treatment of his or her personal records, and the right to approve or refuse the release of these records to any individual outside the facility, except upon transfer to another adult care facility or a nursing home, residential care facility, home for the aging, hospital, or other healthcare facility or provider, and except as required by law or rule or as required by a third-party payment contract.

- The right to be informed in writing of the rates charged by the facility as well as any additional charges, and to receive thirty days' notice in writing of any change in the rates and charges.

- The right to have any significant change in his or her health reported to his or her sponsor.

- The right to share a room with a spouse, if both are residents of the facility.

- The right not to be locked out of the facility. If the facility is locked during any portion of the day, each resident shall be provided with a key or a staff member shall be immediately available on the premises to open the door.

- The right not to be locked in the facility at any time for any reason. All lockable doors shall be capable of being opened by residents from the inside without using a key.

- The right not to be isolated or to have food or other services withheld for punishment, incentive, or convenience.

Unfortunately, the rights of vulnerable people become meaningless if there is lack of enforcement. ACF operators who fail to meet minimum standards are seldom penalized.

EMPLOYMENT AND DISABILITY

Most people retain work capacity even after the onset of serious illness. People who maintain a connection to employment seldom surrender to the mindset of helplessness and dependency. Believing that you have no employment options feeds the pathology of depression and delusion.

Disability is a technical and legal term. Do not give it too much power. Most of the time it simply means that a medical condition has come into play.

MAINTAINING EMPLOYMENT

People with mental illness benefit greatly from continued employment. The symptoms may be disruptive, but if they can be managed, the prospects for long-term recovery improve.

Many people with mental illness keep their jobs. They may take sick leave or vacation, or even unpaid time off while symptoms are at their peak, but they never disconnect from the workforce. If they cannot handle the stress of their current job, they take stock of their capacities, get the support they need, and find a different line of work that they can handle. Make necessary career changes to keep connected to employment. People find new jobs all the time, even when the economy is tough.

EMPLOYMENT DISCRIMINATION

The Americans with Disabilities Act protects people with mental health disabilities from discrimination in employment. Employers are required to make reasonable accommodations that are necessary for a person to perform the essential components of a job. Consult an attorney or the local office of the Equal Employment Opportunity Commission for more information.

VOCATIONAL REHABILITATION

Every state has a vocational rehabilitation services agency that helps people with disabilities get jobs.

Vocational rehabilitation is designed to professionally assess a person's capacities, and supply the education, equipment, and other services that make it possible to rejoin the workforce. Most people with disabilities qualify for an assessment and a plan for employment. The vocational rehabilitation agency can pay for continuing education or specialized job training, supplies and books, work adjustment training, tools and equipment, on-the-job training, and job placement plus follow-up.

Eligibility for services is based on three factors. The person must have a physical, mental, or emotional impairment that creates or results in a substantial barrier to employment. The person must be able to benefit from vocational rehabilitation services in terms of employment outcome. The person must require services to prepare for, enter, engage in, or retain gainful employment.

People applying for services should bring available copies of hospital records and other medical records. Vocational rehabilitation counselors will use these records to build a file that shows that the person is eligible for services. Bringing this information to the first appointment can help streamline the administrative process. The agency will pay for additional testing that is needed to put together an effective rehabilitation plan.

Counseling is provided throughout the process. A successful rehabilitation may take anywhere from several months to several years. Vocational rehabilitation counselors and other staff may connect clients to employers, or help with the job search process.

Vocational rehabilitation offices, like most public agencies, have established timeframes and requirements that can result in sanctions and denials of benefits. An advocate or family member can help clients respond to the agency's various technical requirements.

DISABILITY BENEFITS

Severe mental illness can wipe out a person's capacity to maintain substantial employment. People unable to work for a year or more can become eligible for public benefits. Supplemental Security Income (SSI) and Social Security Disability Insurance (SSDI) are the two primary income programs for people with disabilities. Both are federal programs administered by the Social Security Administration. The programs differ in significant ways. Each has complex legal requirements and complicated procedures that have been shaped by public debate, legislation, and litigation over the course of 75 years or more. The material in this chapter, and even Social Security's own public information materials, covers only a tiny percentage of this subject.

Social Security Disability Insurance (SSDI) is based on an insurance model. The SSDI payment amount is based on a worker's lifetime average earnings covered by Social Security. The average payment to a disabled worker in 2014 is $1,148 per month. If a disabled worker has a qualifying spouse and children, the family can receive an additional 50 to 80 percent of a worker's benefit. Remember, these are averages. Actual payments can be much higher or lower. Unlike SSI, the amount of an SSDI payment is generally not affected by the amount of other income or savings a person has. Earnings from employment do affect benefits.

Supplemental Security Income (SSI) is available only to people with very limited income and resources. The SSI payment amount is based on the amount of other income the person receives, as well as the person's living arrangement. In 2014, the federal SSI payment for an individual living alone is $721 per month. Recipients living in another person's household receive a reduced payment of $480. People living in certain Medicaid-paid institutional arrangements receive only $30 per month. Some states add funding that increases SSI payments.

The process of establishing eligibility for public disability benefits is challenging, complicated and

technical. Dealing with Social Security can be stressful, even intimidating.

Establishing disability is an important threshold
that sets up a connection with Medicare and Medicaid. The amount of a person's check is a second process. Many people who have established eligibility do
not receive a payment. Approval of a disability claim
can validate a person's self-image, and helps many
people come to terms with the effect of an illness.

Get help from an attorney or community agency
early in the application process. Each state has a
network of advisory groups to provide information
and advocacy services to people with disabilities.
Type "disability advocates" plus the name of your
state in an internet search box to connect with these
services.

Do not abandon a Social Security or SSI application once it is filed, even if the claim is denied. Use
the appeal process. Social Security restricts the deci-
sion-making authority of workers in the early stages
of the process. If an application is turned down, the
best chance for benefits is to appeal.

Social Security's disability rules apply to both SSI
and SSDI. These differ from rules of other agencies,
such as worker's compensation. The Social Security
Administration is not required to accept your doctor's
or another agency's diagnosis or evaluation. Even if
your doctor states that you are disabled, or if you are
receiving disability benefits from another organization, you may still not qualify for SSI or SSDI.

Claimants must demonstrate that their medical
condition prevents them from doing any kind of sub-

stantial gainful work. For 2014, this means work that is valued at $1070 per month or more. People who are blind or visually impaired have higher earnings limits. These amounts change slightly every year.

To be eligible for Social Security Disability Insurance (SSDI), a person must have worked and paid Social Security taxes long enough to be covered by Social Security. Some of the taxes must have been paid in recent years. The person must be considered medically disabled, and not working, or working but earning less than the substantial gainful activity limit.

To be eligible for SSI, a person must have little or no income or financial resources, be considered medically disabled, and not working, or working but earning less than the substantial gainful activity limit.

Resources (meaning assets or things people own) or income (money or support a person receives in cash or in kind) over certain set amounts may make the person ineligible for SSI. For example, if friends or family members give gifts of cash, food, or clothing, assist with shelter, or provide any of these things through a will or estate, the person's SSI may be reduced. Similarly, if a person has countable assets totaling over $2000, the person will not be eligible for SSI. For a couple, the resource limit is $3000. Not every asset counts as a resource for SSI purposes.

The SSI resource and income rules are very technical. Friends and relatives can substantially improve an SSI beneficiary's living conditions by knowing the rules and contributing money in ways that do not reduce the amount of the person's payment. For example, giving someone money counts as income, reducing a person's SSI check by the amount of the gift. However, paying vendors directly might not count as income and would not reduce benefits at all. Timing of gifts can also be an important issue. Factors like these are written out in administrative regulations or based in case law. Planning how to use the rules to maximize benefits is legal and makes sense. It is important to get legal advice, understand eligibility rules, and communicate precisely with Social Security workers.

People who receive incorrect benefits will have future benefits adjusted down until money is repaid. Social Security's publications and information materials reflect a punitive administrative mindset with respect to events that cause overpayment of benefits. Get prompt legal advice if you face a potential reduction in benefits.

OTHER SOCIAL SECURITY BENEFITS

There are several categories of Social Security benefits available based on relationship to a person who is either retired, receiving disability, or deceased.

A spouse must be 62 or older, or any age if caring for a disabled child who is receiving Social Security. Divorced spouses may also qualify for benefits. A child must be unmarried, and be under age 18, or be 18-19 years old and a full-time student (no higher than grade 12), or be 18 or older and disabled from a disability that started before age 22.

Benefits are also available to surviving widows and children of workers with enough earnings under Social Security. A widow or widower who has not remarried can receive full benefits at full retirement age or older or reduced benefits as early as age 60. Disabled widows or widowers can begin receiving benefits as early as age 50. Divorced widows or widowers may also qualify for benefits. Children of deceased workers also qualify for benefits. A child must be unmarried and be under age 18, or be 18-19 years old and a full-time student (no higher than grade 12), or be 18 or older and disabled from a disability that started before age 22. Parents of deceased workers may also qualify for benefits.

APPLICATION PROCESS

You should apply for benefits at your local Social Security office as soon as you are eligible. The address and phone number are listed in the telephone directory under U.S. Government, or you can call the national toll-free number, 1-800-772-1213, and they will set up an appointment for you.

The Social Security office will tell you to bring a number of documents to your appointment. The ones you will need depend on the circumstances of your claim, but usually include your Social Security card or number, birth certificate, proof of citizenship, and, if you are employed, a W-2 form or tax return.

Social Security may also request information about any sources of financial support and a list of doctors, hospitals, or clinics where your diagnosis and treatment were received. You should be prepared to discuss your employment in the past 15 years. For SSI, you will need a list of your assets including cash, real estate, and bank accounts. Your home and personal belongings, and usually your car, are not counted as assets.

If you are denied benefits, you may appeal. If you are still denied benefits after each step of the appeals process you may move to the next step, as follows. (1) Ask the local office for a reconsideration of the ruling. (2) Request a hearing before an administrative law judge. (3) Request a review by Social Security's appeals council. (4) Bring a civil suit in federal court.

If you believe you have a valid claim for benefits, it is critical that you continue to pursue your appeals. Social Security restricts the ability of decision makers to approve claims at the first stages of its process. Later in the appeals process you may reach a person with the authority to render a favorable decision.

An attorney familiar with Social Security law can help with your claim by organizing and presenting the evidence in your case, and advocating on your behalf throughout the claims and appeals process. You are permitted to have an attorney or other person represent you in your claim for benefits. The amount of fees an attorney can charge is regulated by the Social Security Administration.

REPRESENTATIVE PAYEES

Some people who receive SSI or SSDI benefits are not able to manage their finances. In those cases, the Social Security office may appoint a friend, relative, or other person to handle the SSI or SSDI benefits. Some people prefer to have their representative payee be someone who works for a local social service organization.

Although the benefits check is made payable to the representative payee, the payee must use the money for the personal care and well-being of the person entitled to benefits. If there is any extra money after bills are paid it must be saved for future needs. The relationship between beneficiary and representative payee can be formal or informal. It is not unusual for payees to set up an allowance that the person with the illness is capable of managing wisely. Payees must be able to account for how they handled funds.

WORK AND BENEFITS

People who have been certified eligible for SSI or SSDI are allowed to work (within certain limits) without losing benefits. However, if they exceed the earnings limit they could lose their SSI or SSDI income and Medicaid or Medicare. It is important to know the differences between SSI and SSDI regulations governing the effect of work and income. Be cautious. Always get advice before returning to work. Know the effect it will have on benefits. People who receive incorrect benefits will have future benefits adjusted down until money is repaid. Social Security's publications and information materials reflect a punitive administrative mindset with respect to events that cause overpayment of benefits. Get prompt legal advice if you face a potential reduction in benefits.

Impact of earnings on SSI benefits. The first $85 of earned income is not counted at all. From $86 of earnings on up, $1 is deducted from the SSI check for every $2 earned. In other words, one-half of the amount earned is later deducted from the amount of the SSI check. Certain work-related expenses may also be deducted before income is counted against the SSI check. If deductions from monthly earnings push over the benefit ceiling and benefits stop they will be started again for any month during the next year that income falls below the ceiling. Medicaid coverage continues, even after SSI benefits stop, until earnings reach a high monthly level. The other conditions for continuation of Medicaid are that (1) it is needed for work, (2) similar private coverage is unaffordable, (3) the disability continues.

Returning to work. Many people with disabilities would like to work but are afraid to try because of concern that their benefits might stop, especially their insurance. The trial work period lets people test their ability to work or run a business for nine months, sometimes more, without affecting their disability benefits. After nine months, Social Security will review the work. If they decide it has been substantial gainful activity (generally, earnings over $1070) benefits will continue for three more months and then stop. Medicare coverage will continue for the entire nine months and then at least 39 months beyond that. Usually, if average monthly earnings are less than $1070, benefits will continue indefinitely. When figuring out whether income has reached $1070, any expenses necessary to working may be deducted, including prescription medications, some transportation, a personal attendant or job coach, or equipment.

Plans for achieving self-support (PASS) can help people receiving SSI accumulate income and/or resources to help achieve a work goal. Under a PASS, funds set aside for work goals are not counted against SSI benefits or program eligibility. PASS set-aside funds can only be used to achieve the vocationally oriented goals of the PASS, not for expansion of general living income. The plan must be documented and monitored in Social Security's files.

The Ticket to Work Act is an attempt to overhaul the interaction between work and federal benefits. Most SSDI and SSI beneficiaries can receive a "ticket" they may use to obtain vocational rehabilitation, employment or other support services from an approved provider to help them go to work and achieve their employment goals. The law also expanded Medicare coverage to people with disabilities who work. Each state has a designated agency to provide Ticket to Work Act services.

WILLS AND ESTATE PLANNING

It is very important for the family to plan so that people receiving SSI payments and Medicaid do not lose benefits or eligibility through inadequate estate planning.

Inheriting property or money can disqualify a person from eligibility for SSI and Medicaid. Usually the inheritance comes from a parent or well-intentioned grandparent. However, it would take a very large inheritance to provide health insurance (if any insurance company would ever insure the person in the first place), support services, or room and board for a person with mental illness who is unable to work.

A lawyer with expertise in Medicaid issues (sometimes called "Elder Law") should be consulted whenever a bequest or inheritance is planned for a person receiving public benefits. The right techniques can ensure that the person receives the full benefit of the intended gift.

PLANNED LIFETIME ASSISTANCE NETWORK

Local Planned Lifetime Assistance Network (PLAN) offices can help families and friends arrange future care for people with disabilities. PLAN assists by setting up a service plan that maintains continued care and supervision of the disabled person.

PLAN provides services that help individuals become more self-sufficient and enhance the quality of life. This can vary from appointment of a representative payee to help with management of finances, to simply being there as a friend or companion, from encouraging or assisting in a crisis to helping learn living skills or finding suitable housing.

A PLAN Family Advocate will guide the person needing care in organizing daily chores, recreational activities, and living and financial arrangements. This professional will also help in preparing the personal plan of care according to the needs of the family, the person needing care, and/or guardian. The overall direction of each PLAN is determined by a volunteer board of directors composed of people receiving services as well as family members. The Board meets regularly to make sure that the quality of services provided by each PLAN is the best and most relevant. Any family that receives services from PLAN may participate in board activities.

It is crucial to the PLAN organization that the person needing care lives as independently as possible and, as the direct result of carefully planned arrangements, lives a life of quality. An important feature of PLAN is to advocate bridging any gaps that may exist between the family, community service agencies, and the person with the disability.

PLAN staff and family members work together to determine needs and resources, and to develop a Personal Plan of Care. Services may vary somewhat from PLAN to PLAN, but in general, services which families want to utilize right away include regular personal contact, transportation, liaison with family, client, and/or community services and agencies, monitoring to assure continuation of benefits, representative payee, money management, household and personal shopping, prevention or resolution of a crisis or legal difficulty.

Enrollment in PLAN does not jeopardize current government benefits such as SSI or Medicaid. PLAN helps families anticipate a person's future needs, and aims to provide a comprehensive care plan throughout the life of the person receiving services. This includes financial and estate planning to insure that the individual continues to receive public benefits and entitlements.

Find the PLAN group in your community by typing "planned lifetime assistance network" in an internet search box.

PART FOUR
NEAR-TERM AND LONG-TERM

SUICIDE PREVENTION

Suicide is a tragic public health problem. About 38,000 people die by suicide in the United States each year. This means, on average, one suicide death every 14 minutes, 104 suicide deaths each day. More than four times as many men as women die by suicide, although women report attempting suicide about three times as often as men do. Suicide is the third leading cause of death among youth aged 15 to 24. Older Americans are also disproportionately likely to die by suicide.

Although there is a close association between mental illness and suicide, a formal diagnosis is not a prerequisite. Effectively reducing the immediate risk of suicide generally involves eliminating access to potential instruments of harm, together with treatment that addresses the person's mental distress. Every state has procedures for providing this treatment, whether or not the person consents.

Suicide risk involves three factors:

1. Thwarted belongingness.

A perception, belief, or feeling of disconnection or alienation from others.

2. Thwarted effectiveness.

A perception, belief, or feeling of failure or worthlessness, or that one has become a burden on others.

3. Acquired capacity for self-harm.

A kind of fearlessness, recklessness, or immunity to pain, which is gained through experience of painful injury, prior self-harm, or through practice of another sort.

Suicide and suicidal behavior are relatively rare. We have all been hurt. Everyone experiences loneliness or failure, yet very few of us ever act on thoughts of self-harm. Even people with elevated risk, those who have acquired the capacity for self-harm, rarely act on their suicidal impulses. People understand that perceptions can be mistaken, that life has value, and that the difficulties they face may be necessary for growth and progress. People realize that distress and trouble are just part of the human condition.

Once a person gains the capacity for self-harm, it is difficult to lose it. Restoring safety typically involves the other main suicide factors. Effective treatment reduces the pain, anxiety and repetitive thought patterns of sadness, failure, and worthlessness caused by depression or other medical issues. Thwarted belongingness and perceived burdensomeness respond to cognitive-behavioral therapy and the actual love and support of friends and family.

People in distress need to hear that their feelings of disconnection and burdensomeness are mistaken. They also need to recognize that they have options. People try to resist thoughts of suicide, and will usually choose alternative courses of action if they recognize that options exist. When tunnel vision takes over, and the person is stuck focusing tightly on relief of immediate overwhelming pain and distress, the person is at grave risk.

When people are experiencing a suicidal crisis, they lose cognitive capacity, especially the ability to generate or recognize options. At this point, people may need a safe environment and close observation.

Suicide risk assessment is difficult, even for experienced clinicians. It is always hard to discern what another person's intentions and capacity might be, let alone the secret story another person is living out. Most people are resilient enough not to attempt a self-destructive act when affected by a stressful event or a troubling emotional state. However, when resiliency is weakened, a triggering event can push a person towards suicidal action. People who have ever "crossed thresholds" (for example by previously attempting suicide) are at the highest risk. Moreover, if people have access to weapons or other deadly means, suicide can happen fast.

SUICIDE RISK FACTORS

RELATED TO THWARTED BELONGINGNESS AND THWARTED EFFECTIVENESS.

- Depression and other mental disorders, and/or a substance-abuse disorder. More than 90 percent of people who die by suicide have these risk factors. Family history of mental disorder or substance abuse. People with borderline personality disorder experience high levels of alienation and feelings of worthlessness, and have extremely high suicide risk.

- Failed relationships, financial loss, or loss of status. Criminal behavior, impending lengthy incarceration. Other shameful circumstances. Disgrace. Shunning. Bullying. Religious or ideological failure.

- Disability, aging, loss of autonomy. Reduced capacity for self-care. Inability to ensure safety of a dependent spouse or disabled adult child.

- Cognitive distortions, delusions, paranoia, rage.

- Frequent nightmares, lack of sleep.

RELATED TO ACQUIRED CAPACITY FOR SELF-HARM.

- Prior suicide attempt (puts the person at highest level of risk).

- Exposure to the suicidal behavior of others, such as family members, peers, or media figures.

- Exposure to violence, including physical or sexual abuse. Exposure to the violent behavior of others. Family violence. Occupational violence, especially for public safety workers. Combat violence. Incarceration.

- Pain and injury, especially self-injury. Multiple surgeries. Frequent tattoos and piercings.

- Risky and reckless behavior, provocative experiences. Disruptive behavior.

- Substance abuse.

- Medication misuse.

- Firearms in the home (the method used in more than half of suicides). Firearms, suffocation, and poisoning are the most frequent means used to commit suicide.

- Vicarious experiences. Opportunities to practice, plan and contemplate self-harm. Violent media, video games.

- Changes in mental health medication. People may become activated as medication takes effect or wears off.

Notice how common and ordinary many of these factors are. It is impossible to remove or eliminate every risk factor for suicide. Nevertheless, we can recognize situations developing and take appropriate action, especially if we learn to spot signs and leaked signals of distress and alienation accumulating around the people we care about.

We can also learn to foster resiliency. The Developmental Assets theory developed by the Search Institute is what YMCA, 4-H, Boys and Girls Clubs and other youth development programs use to build resiliency for their participants. Developmental assets is the term Search Institute uses to describe protective factors like success in school, positive environments, and supportive friendships. The more of these factors a person has in their life, the greater the chances for success, and the smaller the risk of succumbing to dangerous, risky behavior.

SUICIDE PREVENTION SCREENING

It may be difficult to estimate a person's potential for suicide, but it is critical to get it right. Suicide is such a rare event, yet so tragic when it happens. Information about the experiences and intentions of the person involved may be difficult to obtain. People are reluctant to disclose what they are experiencing, or to express their intentions directly. They may try to hide their intentions, but might speak out indirectly, or act in ways that signal trouble.

High-risk environments (institutions like jails, prisons, and hospitals) use suicide prevention screening protocols that rely on statistical methods and objective factors. The most effective screening protocols require action whether or not the person in question has verbalized that they are suicidal. The score on the screening instrument determines what happens next. If the screening tool indicates high risk, people take action. For example, people entering jails facing certain types of criminal charges are routinely placed under suicide watch. Suicide watch involves frequent or constant close observation of the person.

Primary care physicians are increasingly required to screen for suicidality. Older adults as well as women who die by suicide are likely to have seen a primary care provider in the year prior to their suicide. Because high-risk patients seldom bring up suicide or depression at these doctor visits, doctors initiate these screenings whether or not the person brings the topic up.

Unfortunately, at the threshold of a hospital or a hospital emergency room, professionals must deal both with the actual potential for suicide, and with the capacity of the institution to do something about it. If hospitals have few beds available for new patients, or if resources to deliver a safe environment are lacking, clinical standards can slip. It becomes more likely that ambiguous signals about suicide risk will be discounted. Many tragic incidents occur when people at moderate to high risk of suicide are sent home by hospital personnel without a plan in place for personal support or safety.

WHAT ORDINARY PEOPLE CAN DO

Family, friends, co-workers, and neighbors are the heart of suicide prevention. Emergency responders cannot act unless the risk is immediate and serious. Police or a crisis team might be able to make a safety visit, but even if that happens, people need the support of friend and family members to stay safe.

Anyone can learn how to have the right kind of chat with a person we think is in trouble. We might prefer to give this task over to a professional, but that is not always possible and might not happen in time. Anyway, we are closest to the people we love. We may never know the difference our actions might make.

Here is a little script, just four questions anyone can use to screen for trouble. Try to have a brief chat in a public place but out of earshot of other people. Ask the following questions one at a time, in order. Practice the questions out loud. Yes, this is awkward. You can use your own words, but follow the pattern. Listen to the person's answer. People benefit simply by knowing they have been heard.

1. What have you accomplished since the last time we talked?

2. What are you facing?

3. Who are your allies?

4. What is your plan?

As you listen, be on the lookout for suicide risk factors. These include extreme discouragement or recent shameful loss, no ability to make effective plans, prior suicide attempts or violence, substance abuse, a failure of addiction or mental health treatment, difficulty verbally expressing feelings, stress, trouble relating to other people's feelings, the onset of schizophrenia or another major mental illness, and lack of sources of support.

If you start to feel worried, help connect your friend to a more formal source of help. You may have the single most important opportunity to help your friend. If you detect tunnel vision and a sense of diminishing options, or the person talks about suicide, or expresses a lack of hope or a feeling that they are a burden, or cannot respond meaningfully, ask the person directly about thoughts of suicide. Suicide is much more likely than violence directed against other people. Ask directly using these words: "Are you thinking about killing yourself?"

If you sense that the person is becoming suicidal, stay with the person. Try to persuade them to seek help from their doctor or visit an emergency room. Offer to help them get in contact with a crisis hotline by calling 1-800-273-8255 or dialing 911. Help them scribble down a quick plan to get through the next few days.

People who are suicidal should not be left alone. Check on them if they get up at night. It is also important to limit the person's access to firearms, medications, or other lethal methods for suicide. Since suicide is more likely to occur if the individual is under the influence of alcohol or street drugs, these should also be taken away or minimized.

Hospitals have trained staff, facilities, and procedures that can keep a person safe. If a person refuses voluntary treatment, investigate the requirements for involuntary hospitalization. The course of treatment involves close monitoring, plus medication, plus on-going talk therapy. Most people respond to treatment in a relatively short time, perhaps a few days, sometimes a few weeks. In 2010, the average length of a hospital stay for a mental health concern was 7.2 days.

Some people do resist evaluation and treatment. This becomes less of a problem when people trust their friends and family. Personal connections help people learn how treatment helps them reach a healthy emotional state with the ability to concentrate and a stable sleep pattern. People who realize they need hospital care from time to time make contingency plans that address this.

Caregivers need to address their own challenges. Providing care and handling events at home, let alone dealing with a suicidal person, is difficult and emotionally draining. NAMI and Mental Health America offer caregiver education and support.

Community organizations and many churches also sponsor caregiver support groups.

Suicide prevention training is available through the QPR Institute at www.qprinstitute.com/ and from many community groups.

Suicide is a frightening and horrible event that shakes up not only the family, but everyone who knew the individual. Nonetheless, family members must realize that just as we cannot always save family members from accidents or disease, we cannot always save them from suicide.

IF YOU FEEL SUICIDAL

If you are feeling suicidal, call your doctor or call the crisis hotline 1-800-273-8255. The national suicide prevention lifeline is a national, federally funded network of local crisis centers providing suicide prevention and intervention services through this toll-free telephone number. In most communities, you can also call 911 to reach a crisis line. Ask someone to remain with you and help you stay safe.

For ongoing support when the crisis has passed, talk with a family member, a friend or a community support program worker.

Above all, do not isolate yourself. As difficult as it may be, try to get out of the house or apartment. Thoughts can become obsessive if you spend too much time alone, and it is hard to break out of a pattern of thinking. Try to engage in activities you enjoy as much as you can.

Listening to others helps generate options. It may help to join a support group. The shared experience of people in your group can show you that the pain you are experiencing does not go on with such intensity forever. When we are in too much pain, we tend not to think objectively. This creates blind spots and tunnel vision. We fail to consider all the options and fail to evaluate consequences properly. Other people's input can help us get rid of our tunnel vision, our tendency to focus on getting rid of the pain. Rage and anger (often turned inward) will dominate a suicidal mood. It is especially important to talk to people who can help you get a healthier perspective.

Cognitive behavioral therapy can improve distressing thought patterns. Writing thoughts down on paper or making positive plans sometimes helps. Reading affirmative and inspirational books helps some people. Other people find that meditation, prayer, or talking to their pastor or rabbi helps them through tough spots.

Remember, depressions lift. People find that life is worth living again. However, these things are difficult to accomplish alone. You must reach out for help.

CRISIS AND ESCALATION

The connection between mental illness and violence is weaker than we tend to think. Most people with mental illness are far more likely to be victimized. In fact, most people with a mental health diagnosis suffer quietly, never reaching a crisis point.

However, mental health crisis does occur, and when it occurs it can be terrifying. Risk of harm increases as self-control and reality-based thinking deteriorate. This risk endures throughout the crisis until it completely resolves.

More knowledge about mental health crisis can help keep people safe. Knowledgeable people can anticipate what will happen, and help keep situations from spinning out of control. Unfortunately, our culture (and the innate human tendency to avoid trouble) keeps most of us uninformed, preventing us from being as effective as we might be. We can work on that.

People who have experienced mental health crisis say it is like being stuck in an overwhelming painful loop of difficult thoughts and emotions. There is usually a buildup of tension. The buildup can be long or short. The situation eventually accelerates and gains intensity. People speak of being overcome, feeling frustrated, disconnected, losing time, being pushed into some action. Stress hormones are working. People experience the fight-or-flight response.

The notion of "multiple intelligences" and the enormous variety of human talents continue to play out during a crisis. Even when self-control deteriorates, even when agitation increases, and even when someone experiences delusions or hallucinations, the person retains other cognitive and noncognitive capacities. The capacities that the person retains might be the starting points for de-escalation, or might enhance potential danger. Some people can carry out elaborate plans while hiding their intentions, even while experiencing delusions.

What happens during a crisis differs from incident to incident and from one person to the next. One person may become overemotional; another might pace and shout; a third might have a tantrum; a fourth might threaten someone; a fifth might hurt himself; a sixth might attack someone.

The best indication of what might happen is what the person has experienced before. However, it is not safe to rely solely on prior experience. Do not write off or underestimate the potential danger building up around a person who is losing control. Learn to assess what is happening, and be mindful of your own safety. Be cautious. Anyone, even experienced law enforcement officers, can become seriously injured or even die during the course of a mental health crisis incident.

CRISIS PREVENTION STRATEGIES

Effective long-term crisis prevention for most people with mental illness means controlling the internal noise level by managing symptoms, plus controlling the stress factors within the environment, plus building self-management skills. As the person builds impulse control and self-manages symptoms, the risk of violent action goes down.

It is good practice to make a psychiatric emergency contingency plan. Call the local NAMI affiliate or local psychiatric emergency room for details on what ordinarily takes place in your community when people experience a mental health crisis. There may be a mobile crisis team or crisis hotline you can call.

SAFER BY DESIGN

Safety begins far in advance of an incident, with a responsive, positive home life, and an environment that reduces risk.

- Heavy furniture that is difficult to pick up or throw.

- No weapons.

- No candles, open flames, or smoking.

- No chemicals that pose a risk to health.

- A sleeping area that affords privacy but does not include televisions, computers, or other "screens."

- Mobile phones are turned off overnight, and recharged outside of the bedroom.

- A cleaning and maintenance routine that includes screening for contraband.

- An alcohol-free home.

- An emphasis on pro-social media.

Above all, safety comes from reduced frustration and a positive, meaningful life. People need experiences that help them feel connected, capable, and safe. Make a list of what helps anyone feel safe, productive, and normal.

- Activities and a social life in ordinary places everyone enjoys.

- Work, or productive activities that we choose

- The opportunity to do what we are good at, and accomplish something

- Love, family, and relationships.

- Good health

- Spirituality or a sense of purpose.

It is normal to want to protect a person, but it is a mistake to think that restricting a person's freedom increases safety. In institutions, activity restrictions and scheduling demands create conflict and cause violent incidents to break out. In communities, it makes sense to pay attention to the level of stimulation that can be tolerated. This helps us learn to self-manage exposure to stress.

TIMING ISSUES AND RISK

People with high volatility are sometimes safer at certain times of the day or month. People might do better earlier in the day, when they are rested, and worse later on, after a day of coping with stress or managing frustrations. Small yet predictable annoyances also wear on people. In residential programs, incidents tend to cluster around times when people must respond to institutional demands, like scheduled times for taking medication. In schools, incidents might tend to cluster around transitions or around times when there is less control over what other students are doing.

HANDLING CRISIS SITUATIONS

When an emergency hits, call the mental health emergency number or dial 911. Dispatchers are trained to handle calls involving mental illness. Follow the dispatcher's instructions.

STAGES OF ESCALATION

There is a pattern to incidents fueled by anger and frustration. These few paragraphs merely identify the stages. The material that follows is adapted from Kevin Fateux's book *Defusing Angry People*. This is only the escalation part of the equation. It takes study and practice to develop effective de-escalation skills. Escalation can happen slow or fast. People who must deal with volatile situations learn to identify incidents as they begin to emerge, and respond quickly to defuse them.

STAGE ONE. LISTENING TO FRUSTRATION

The person is feeling denied or disrespected, or in some way slighted. His focus is on the situation, not you. The person needs to stand up for himself and be heard.

STAGE TWO. DEFENSIVE ANGER

At this stage, anger expresses not only the frustration of being disrespected or ignored but also the emotional hurt that comes from it. Humiliation and failure. The anger protects the person from feeling vulnerable.

STAGE THREE. DIFFICULT ANGRY PEOPLE

People who are chronically argumentative, abrasive, opinionated, and obstinate use situations as a way of "standing up to you" in order to keep an emotional distance. The situation is a way to test your limits. The person is goal-oriented, less emotional. What you see is classic passive/aggressive behavior. The person is uncooperative, instead of expressive and direct. For someone who is oppositional and defiant, everything becomes a contest.

STAGE FOUR. HOSTILITY

Events at this stage have moved beyond frustration to intense expression of hostility, anger that is aggressively aimed at you. More adrenaline is pumping. People are moving towards a fight. Verbal attacks are no longer focused on the situation, but aimed at you. The goal is intimidation. There is a malicious or menacing quality. The person blames you for his humiliation or peril. He uses this to try to manipulate you. Physical signs include clenched fist, vicious stare, belligerent stance, sweaty, wringing hands, and clenched jaw.

STAGE FIVE. RAGE

At this point, there is not only an expression of anger, but also loss of control. The person may have trouble controlling impulses, a short fuse. A regressive temper tantrum may come with little warning. Rage is not manipulative. It is simply a feeling of being overwhelmed and out of control. Some people enjoy this feeling, and can become addicted to rage.

STAGE SIX. THREATS

Some people become enraged and lose control of their anger. Others make threats in order to control you. This is a crisis. Anger makes the person stand up to tower over you in order to threaten physically to push you around. Warning signs a threat is real: The person blames you; perceives threats as only choice; threatens obsessively; expresses agitated body language; presents a plan to harm; has a predisposition to violence; disregards warnings; is under the influence of alcohol or drugs. Threats that are concrete and specific are the most dangerous. Other dangerous threats can involve a gesture or movement; acting as if violence is justifiable now that you have failed to deliver; saying "I don't care who you call" or "bring them on. I'm ready;" and paranoid thinking. "I know you are out to get me."

Sociopaths have a deeply ingrained predisposition to approaching problems with threats and violence. Antisocial, manipulative, vengeful, pathological liars lack regard for others or for the consequences of their actions. Relations are one-sided, "with me or against me." Violent people may be **psychopathic** too. Unemotional, paranoid, aggressively impulsive, with an inflated sense of superiority. Sociopaths have no morals. Grandiosity makes him right and you wrong. He is not swayed by consequences. May not appear angry, uses charm to get his goal. Trusts no one. Thrill-seeking. Enjoys frightening you. Likes being perceived as dangerous. Deals out cold-blooded vengeance – does not follow the usual escalation pattern.

Psychosis. "God told me to kill you if you don't do as I say." An interruption in medication increases risk of violence.

Substance abuse and aggression. Alcohol leads to greater impulsivity plus cognitive impairment. It disinhibits people, and makes people feel entitled to act recklessly and irresponsibly. People can become enraged. **Amphetamines and cocaine** increase energy, give a feeling of power and physical strength, but they also makes a person anxious, paranoid, hyperactive, impatient, irrational, even psychotic. A concrete weapon plus paranoia makes a threat very serious. For **heroin and opiates**, the danger comes at withdrawal, with frantic drug-seeking , obsessive even threatening behavior focused on getting a fix. With **marijuana**, excessive amounts of THC can lead to aggressive behavior. **Inhalants** can cause brain damage that can lead to aggressive behavior. Steroids – can lead to intense anger ("roid rage").

STAGE SEVEN. VIOLENCE

Anger and aggression, abetted by anxiety, accelerate into assault. You are pushed, punched, slapped, kicked, bludgeoned, stabbed, or shot. Anger is used to knock you down. It is the time of action. Violence usually has a goal, to get what the person wants when nothing else including threats would procure it. Sometimes there is no warning. Sometimes the person blames you for "making him resort to violence." Aggressors sometimes "even the score," punishing you for pushing him to his limit or making him lose face or humiliating him.

POST-ASSAULT. DEBRIEFING

You must process the trauma of the experience. You can take action that will improve the next time you face such a situation.

HELPING A FRIEND THROUGH A CRISIS

Note: The information here is for people who find themselves with an opportunity to help someone that they know. Always arrange back-up. Always call emergency services if the situation appears dangerous. Never enter a situation involving a person with a weapon.

For people who are neither clinicians nor law enforcement, the key tools of de-escalation are safe environments, relationships, stress reduction, time, space, and listening. Family members and friends often have the best opportunity to prevent incidents from escalating. Above all, friends and family can listen to their friend or relative's concerns, and ally themselves with the person's hopes and dreams. But even this may not be enough to eliminate every incident. Friends and family are often the first to learn of a developing incident. They arrive as the incident develops, and they have information that is seldom available to public safety workers who arrive at the scene much later.

Always assess the situation before deciding to intervene. There are two parts to this. You must think that you are safe, and you must feel that you are safe. Let the slow part of your brain analyze what is happening. Figuring out the story line that is playing out helps you plan what you might say or do. As you do this, other parts of your brain are working too, reacting to potential threats. Listen to what your body tells you about potential danger. Look at people's hands. Check for potential weapons within reach. Glance at the person who is having the crisis. Listen for threats. What emotions do you see reflected in the person's face and body language? Do not proceed further if you have no plan or feel unsafe.

Enter the situation in a non-threatening manner, hands visible. Greet the person. In a calm, respectful tone of voice, ask what you can do to help.

Tell the others in the room that you need them to give you some space so you can help the person.

Listen to what the person says.

Remain calm. Say "Wow. I hear you. Can I help you figure out what to do?" or say "Wow, I am sorry that happened."

Ask the others in the room to give you some more space so you can help the person. At this point, it may be possible to have others leave the room, and remove objects that could be used as weapons. Explain that you need to make the environment safer so you can concentrate and try to help the person.

Your calm demeanor gives everyone in the room behavior to imitate, a small step towards reducing the stress of the situation. Bystanders can feed negative energy back into disorderly situations, which increases the pressure on the person having the crisis, and makes things worse.

Do not approach the person too closely or back the person into a corner. Freedom of movement is important when the fight or flight response is kicking in.

You may offer the person something to eat.

Be respectful. Resolving the crisis will take time.

Do not try to conquer or overwhelm. Never threaten or attempt to restrain the person. Instead, model calm behavior, and try to provide the structure the person needs until the person can regain control. People in crisis crave stability. When you appear stable, supportive and calm you may be able to provide the structure and control the person needs.

Control the environment while maintaining communications. Do not flee the room if you know you are safe, because of the potential risk of suicide.

Use short, direct, open-ended questions to find out what is happening. Allow the person time to answer each one.

Ask what is troubling the person.

Ask why there is a crisis at this point.

Allow moments of silence to occur. This will show you are not trying to rush the person.

Help the person understand that you are listening. Repeat what the person has told you, and ask if you understood correctly.

Be aware of what is not being said. People in crisis can develop tunnel vision. Help the person become more receptive to exploring options, thinking creatively and solving problems.

Help the person identify personal resources. If you can, help the person see the crisis as a temporary state that can be resolved successfully.

It is vital that you avoid judgments and put-downs. Do not belittle the person. Do not make light of the situation that caused the crisis.

If you cannot make sense of the words the person says, try reacting to the emotional content. Say you understand the person is upset, or frightened. Say you want to help and that you are trying to do what you can.

Ask the person if you can sit with them until more help comes.

Try to stay with the person until help comes, but look out for your own safety. Use all your senses, staying aware of everything that you see, hear, feel, sense, and touch. Trust your instincts about your own personal safety.

Look for warning signs of imminent physical violence: tremor, rigid posture, clenching jaws and fists, pulsing arteries in the temples, verbal abuse and profanity, and hyperactivity. Pre-assault behavior includes verbal abuse, raised voice, swearing, and standing uncomfortably close. Be cautious. Even police officers with specialized crisis intervention training have suffered fatal injuries responding to a mental illness crisis.

After the crisis, make sure to process what happened and debrief. Use your experience to refine your plan for the future.

UNDERSTANDING RISK OF VIOLENCE

A good rule of thumb is that violent people commit violent crimes. Like all Americans, most people with mental health issues are far more likely to be victims of violence than they are to commit violence.

Violence is learned behavior. The vast majority of people who commit violent acts in the community develop the capacity for violence during childhood through a process that involves witnessing violence, experiencing violence, and practicing violence. This changes a person's mental model of the world. Eventually the person regards himself as violent or as capable of doing violence when circumstances warrant. People who have not experienced this type of "violentization" seldom if ever commit serious violence.

Violence, abuse, and trauma in the home result in a brutal social cycle of the strong preying on the weak. Violence researcher Bruce Perry calls this a "vortex of violence."

> The major setting for violence in America is the home. Intrafamilial abuse, neglect and domestic battery account for the majority of physical and emotional violence suffered by children in this country. Despite this, a majority of our

entertainment, media and public policy efforts focus on community or predatory violence. Understanding the roots of community and predatory violence is impossible unless the effects of intra-familial violence and the impact of abuse and neglect on the development of the child are examined. The adolescents and adults responsible for violence in the community developed these violent behaviors as a result of intrafamilial violence during childhood.

Most violence against men is committed by men. Most violence committed against women is committed by men. Most violence against children is committed by women. Most violence committed by children is against other children. Most violence against pets is committed by children.

We usually encounter two types of violence in civilian life: instrumental violence and expressive violence. People with mental illness commit both types.

Instrumental violence is used to gain control over others. This is the violence of robbery and terrorism. People who commit instrumental violence regard themselves as violent, or as willing to do violence if circumstances warrant. Alcohol abuse adds risk by lowering inhibitions. Social and cultural factors can also affect violence risk. For example, people become more violent in the company of other violent people. Communities that have high rates of violence also tend to produce more violence.

There is also some connection between instrumental violence and delusional thinking. A person who experiences delusions may retain the capacity to plan and commit horrible crimes.

The second type of violence, **expressive violence**, is the failure of self-control. People break down and strike out. Anger and frustration builds up to a violent outburst. For people with mental illness, most violence is expressive violence. Handling the internally generated background noise of symptoms is difficult enough. Stress and conflict make the internal noise level worse. The "fight or flight" response kicks in. Nevertheless, people usually do control their behavior, even at this point.

Most people with mental illness never become violent. People with severe mental illness but no substance abuse and no prior violence have a very low probability of becoming violent. However, risk factors pile up. The risk of violence increases if the person has more than one psychiatric disorder. The higher the number of co-occurring psychiatric disorders, the greater the risk of violence. The combination of substance abuse and major mental illness is even more volatile. The most important predictor of future violence is past violence. Risk skyrockets once someone commits their first act of violence. For example, nearly a third of people with schizophrenia also abuse alcohol or drugs. These individuals are, statistically speaking, twice as likely as the average person to become violent. If such a person commits a violent act, the likelihood of future violence doubles yet again.

In community settings, people with paranoid delusions are more violent than people in other mental illness categories. Their violence is well planned, aligned with their delusion, and aimed at individuals or institutions. These individuals are likely to commit the most serious crimes because they can gain access to weapons, stay relatively well connected to reality, and maintain an ability to plan.

There are many other patterns of violence connected with mental illness symptoms. For example, people with depression can react to despair by striking out at other people. Mothers of young children sometimes kill their children when psychotic, or severely depressed, or when contemplating suicide.

Dangerousness involves four factors: magnitude, likelihood, imminence, and frequency. Courts weigh these factors to determine if the facts justify involuntary treatment. Courts will order treatment if a person with mental illness represents a substantial risk of physical harm to others as manifested by evidence of recent homicidal or other violent behavior, evidence of recent threats that place another in reasonable fear of violent behavior and serious physical harm, or other evidence of present dangerousness.

Because everyone's experience of mental illness is so different, it is entirely appropriate to ask treatment providers what risk patterns to look out for. Everyone has a stake in safety. Talking about risk does not make violence happen.

SUICIDE-CONNECTED VIOLENCE

Mass killings like the events in Newtown, Connecticut or the 2012 Sikh Temple shootings are devastating tragic pile-ups. They involve suicidal intent, plus homicidal intent, plus an activating factor, a provocation or a buildup, plus a kind of acquired fearlessness built up through practice or familiarity with violence. The suicide portion of the equation involves both disconnection from others and feelings of thwarted effectiveness. The homicide portion usually connects with revenge violence or the need to make a statement, or to act out a violent fantasy, something the person may have read about or a scene from a movie or a video game. Terrorist suicide bombing cases usually involve a susceptible person pressured towards suicide by political groups. The political group hijacks the susceptible person's suicidal intent and converts it into murder.

Suicide-connected violence is extremely rare. Only 1.7 percent of suicides also involve a homicide. People who commit suicide-homicides are much more like people who commit suicide than they are like people who commit homicides.

For this reason, as they are developing, suicide-homicides and mass killings usually look like the early stages of mental breakdowns and suicides. Clues and hints of distress and trouble accumulate around a person. We might see problems related to how the person is thinking, failure to succeed at work or school, trouble in life, loss of a girlfriend, or other experiences of shame and guilt. We may also notice expressions of hurt or resentment. When a critical point is reached (and sometimes after surprisingly careful planning) the person takes action.

It is in the planning, preparation and action stages where suicides and violent attacks diverge. An attacker strikes out against an institution, person, or group, or even against random people.

Because these incidents often involve suicide warning signals, it is possible to leverage what we understand about suicide prevention to prevent violent incidents. This is an example of a security strategy known as overengineering, giving a system capacity to solve many frequently occurring problems in order to address one large infrequently occurring threat. If more members of the public how to detect, prevent, and interrupt suicides, more violence could be interrupted or prevented. Of course, effective security requires overlapping strategies, so we will still need informants and police. Caution is required. Bystanders or law enforcement personnel can be killed or injured when attempting to intervene in suicide attempts, especially those that involve firearms.

THE PUBLIC'S ROLE IN PREVENTION

Vague, ambiguous signs of trouble show up well ahead of a point of crisis. There may never be enough identifiable risk factors to support a mental health diagnosis. Mental health professionals usually say that violent incidents cannot be predicted, but this may be mere denial. Understanding what risks might be increasing around someone we know is substantially different from predicting random violence in a population through statistics.

Some risk factors are merely circumstantial. We can all recognize times when people benefit from extra support and friendship. For example, returning members of active duty military have higher rates of suicide or domestic violence simply because of the difficult nature of military deployment. Another example: We know how hard it is to deal with the loss of a job. Social support from friends or others in the community may increase resiliency just enough to prevent a person from acting impulsively.

In most of these situations, the only possible intervention is below the level of our formal systems. Prevention is the responsibility of family, friends, coworkers, and neighbors. Even if reported, emergency responders cannot act forcefully if the risk is not immediate and serious. Sometimes the police or a crisis team may be able to make a safety check visit to a person's home.

If there is low risk of imminent trouble, the best thing anyone can do is to support their friend. This helps prevent feeling isolated and helps build resiliency. You are unlikely to ever know if the steps you take to support a friend have prevented a suicide or interrupted a developing course of violence. You want the person to become more resilient and successful, so that the outcome is positive. You want to stay in a position where your relationship permits you to offer more support or call in help when needed.

If you see a neighbor or acquaintance display signs they are encountering problems in their life, you can try the "Four Questions Among Friends" script. The questions are broad enough to help smoke out some signs of trouble, and double as a way of delivering some support. No diagnosis or labeling is involved.

Try to have a brief chat in a public place but out of earshot of other people. Ask these questions one at a time, in order. Practice the questions aloud. We know this is awkward. You can use your own words, but follow the pattern. Listen to the person's answer. People benefit simply by knowing they have been heard.

1. What have you accomplished since the last time we talked?

2. What are you facing?

3. Who are your allies?

4. What is your plan?

As you listen, be on the lookout for risk factors. These include prior violence, substance abuse, a failure of addiction or mental health treatment, difficulty verbally expressing feelings, stress, extreme discouragement or recent shameful loss, no ability to make effective plans, trouble relating to other people's feelings, the onset of schizophrenia or another major mental illness, and lack of sources of support.

If you start to feel worried, offer to connect your friend to a more formal source of help. You may have the single most important opportunity to help your friend. If you detect tunnel vision and a sense of diminishing options, or the person talks about suicide, or expresses a lack of hope, ask the person directly about thoughts of suicide. Suicide is much more likely than violence directed against other people. Ask directly using these words: "Are you thinking about killing yourself?"

If you sense that the person is becoming suicidal, stay with the person. Try to persuade them to seek help from their doctor or visit an emergency room. Offer to help them get in contact with a crisis hotline by calling 1-800-273-8255 or dialing 911.

Effective suicide prevention training is available online through the QPR Institute at www.qprinstitute.com/ and from many community groups.

People with chronic elevated risk of suicide and violence may be appropriate candidates for assertive community treatment or for conservatorship or guardianship. They may need speedy access to hospital treatment. It may be too risky for them to have access to weapons.

Caution: If you ever detect homicidal, vengeful intent, or see evidence of violent plans or preparations, take steps to get to safety and contact law enforcement immediately.

MANAGING CHRONIC VIOLENCE RISK

Violence is learned behavior, and is hard to unlearn. Programs that serve people who have difficulty living peacefully organize the environment and use trained staff to reduce violence risk. Situations involving frustration and anger can usually be de-escalated. Safe environments and appropriate use of de-escalation can completely eliminate the need for restraints and seclusion in schools and treatment programs.

Proper treatment, safe environments, and supportive relationships help people learn to live more peacefully and successfully. Many chronically violent people have cognitive difficulties and trouble managing relationships and emotions. Risk of harm skyrockets when treatment is interrupted or supports fail. Even so, most violent incidents can be interrupted as they develop, especially if the environment can be managed, and if there is sufficient opportunity for the person to regain self-control. People in crisis can be de-escalated before they become a deadly risk. Police Crisis Intervention Teams practice for such situations. This reduces law enforcement injuries as well as injuries to bystanders and people in crisis.

SURVIVING VIOLENT INCIDENTS

The odds of encountering and interrupting a person bent on violence are extremely slim. However, if you ever encounter a true threat, you are likely to feel it instinctively, particularly as you become more aware of risk factors.

Act immediately to stay safe. Do not put yourself in harm's way. If you start to feel worried about accumulating signs of potential violence, find your way to safety, and dial 911. Remember, you are not trained to handle deadly emergencies.

If you are present when a violent attack breaks out, stay low, take cover, and attempt to escape to safety. If escape is not possible, and safe cover is not available, disrupting and overcoming the attacker may be your best option.

INVOLUNTARY HOSPITALIZATION, GUARDIANSHIP AND ALTERNATIVES

Balancing the need for treatment of a very ill person with the individual's civil rights is one of the greatest challenges of commitment law. Involuntary hospitalization is an emergency procedure to be used only when absolutely necessary. All efforts should be made to provide the person with needed services in the community, and when that is impossible, to convince the person to accept hospital treatment voluntarily.

INVOLUNTARY HOSPITALIZATION

Under limited circumstances, a person may need to be involuntarily hospitalized because of the effects of mental illness. Every state has legal procedures that govern these situations. This book presents only the briefest outline of the terms, procedures, and issues involved in the civil process. People with criminal court involvement generally remain subject to the jurisdiction of the criminal court.

The involuntary hospitalization process is typically under the jurisdiction of local Probate Courts. Each local court has rules and forms governing the process. Although court personnel do not give legal advice, they do provide general information about the process in their courts. In addition, many local courts have information about their rules and procedures on their websites.

Note: This process applies only to the person's hospitalization. It does not result in a guardian being appointed for the person. The requirements and procedures for appointing a guardian are covered separately.

Every state has a statute with key definitions that govern the involuntary hospitalization or commitment process. Each stature defines what is considered mental illness. Often this is described as a substantial disorder of thought, mood, perception, orientation, or memory that grossly impairs judgment, behavior, capacity to recognize reality, or ability to meet the ordinary demands of life.

Hospitalization can be ordered where there is substantial risk of physical harm to self or others. The level of required evidence to support the finding is usually very high. Harm to self usually requires evidence of threats of suicide or evidence of suicide attempts or serious self-harm. Harm to others proven with evidence of homicidal or other violent behavior, threats that cause fear of harm to another, or other evidence that the person is presently dangerous. In some states, a person can be hospitalized for injuriousness to self with proof that they are incapable of providing for their basic physical needs because of their mental illness. Evidence of behavior that creates a grave and imminent risk to substantial rights of others may be enough to justify court action.

The evidence must show that a person would benefit from treatment in a hospital for the person's mental illness. If it is determined that the person no longer needs to be involuntarily hospitalized, he must be discharged from the institution.

The involuntary commitment process can begin in several ways. One involves the police. Another involves the county's designated pre-screening mental health agency. The police or the designated agency must agree that the person appears to meet one of the above standards. At this time, the person can be detained at a hospital or crisis center for 72 hours. Then a "probable cause hearing" must take place before a judge. The hospitalized person is represented by counsel at this hearing.

It is important for everyone concerned to get the person's case manager or physician involved. Frequently these professionals will be able to help the person voluntarily seek appropriate treatment. This can spare everyone the ordeal of a final commitment hearing.

The court will order an evaluation to determine if hospitalization is necessary. Family, friends, and clinicians can also provide written or oral testimony to help the court make its determination.

The purpose of the probable cause hearing is to determine whether the person is an appropriate candidate for commitment. As stated above, the person must be mentally ill, a good candidate for treatment, and meet the criterion of dangerousness to self or others.

Many times, the outcome of the probable cause hearing is a settlement agreement, similar to a plea bargain in the criminal justice system. Settlement agreements usually include a formal contract to co-operate with recommended psychiatric treatment, usually for a period of 30, 60 or 90 days. If the person does cooperate, the formal proceedings are dropped.

The final hearing is typically held within 10 calendar days of the emergency detention. The hospitalized person is again represented by counsel. People who know the patient may be asked to testify. The patient is present and may testify. The hospital staff, the police if they were involved, and community treatment agency personnel may testify. Two physicians (or one physician and one psychologist) will discuss the results of the psychiatric examinations.

Courts value family member testimony and participation in the involuntary commitment process. Family members may recognize patterns of behavior that recur when someone is becoming seriously suicidal or completely unable to function outside a protective setting. In many cases, family members also step forward to provide support for the person after hospitalization.

The most effective testimony supporting the need for involuntary hospitalization is specific rather than vague, and points out ways the person's behavior endangers self or others. Some examples follow.

"She sits in her darkened room all day, won't eat a thing except water and fruit. She leaves notes around the house saying she doesn't want to go on living. Here are some of the notes."

"He threw a jar of mayonnaise at me and if I hadn't ducked I might have been seriously hurt. He has done similar things to other family members. He threw a chair at his sister."

"He drives his car recklessly, endangering people, backing out of the driveway without looking, hitting fences and curbs."

Outcomes of the final hearing. After hearing all testimony, the judge makes the final decision. The possible outcomes of a hearing are dismissal, or commitment to the county board of mental health services or its designated agency. If commitment is chosen this usually means that the person will remain in the hospital for a period of time and then receive community services.

Periodic reviews. The court will set a time frame for reviewing the continuing need for involuntary hospitalization, usually at least once per year.

Length of stay. Hospital care is very expensive. It is not unusual for a person to be discharged after a hospital stay of a week or two. The court does not usually need to give permission when a person is discharged.

GUARDIANSHIP

Guardianship will always be controversial.

Guardianship limits a person's right to make decisions about many aspects of life. Everyone should have the right to make their own decisions about their medical treatment and the way they conduct their lives.

However, some people, a small minority of those most severely affected by illnesses such as schizophrenia and bipolar disorder, may not be capable of exercising good judgment, or are not competent to make other decisions. Guardianship may be appropriate for these individuals.

The guardianship process, and many alternatives short of guardianship, can bring relief to people with the most severe illnesses. Still it is important to realize how serious a deprivation of rights occurs when a person is placed under guardianship. That is why, in many states it is possible to limit the extent to which a person's rights are affected. This can be done through a limited guardianship where the guardian has only those powers specifically named by the court order and the ward retains all rights in other areas of life.

RIGHTS TAKEN AWAY IN GUARDIANSHIP

When reviewing the consequences of guardianship, it is best to imagine that you are the ward. If a person is determined by probate court to be totally incompetent and a guardian is appointed for the person and/or estate, then the guardian assumes authority and the ward loses rights in the many areas of ordinary life.

Cannot change residence. You find a nice new apartment, but your guardian will not let you move because you would be farther away from the guardian's home.

Cannot sign a contract. You want to buy a color TV but you cannot sign the contract for a six-month loan.

Cannot withdraw own money. You want to withdraw money from your savings account for Christmas presents, but the bank has been told your guardian must do it.

Cannot sue. The next-door neighbor runs over your bicycle with his van. He does not want an increase in his insurance premiums, so he promises to pay for it himself. That was six months ago. You tell him that you will sue if he does not pay. He laughs and tells you that you cannot sue. He is right. Your guardian must do it for you.

Cannot give or withhold medical consent. You have a mild heart attack. Your doctor tells you if you lose weight, change your eating habits and start a fitness program you probably will do just as well as if you have heart bypass surgery. You want to change your lifestyle, but your guardian wants to play it safe by scheduling surgery. She is afraid you will not lose weight and arranges for the surgery because she is the one who gives medical consent.

Cannot get vocational training. You want to take a course to become a beautician. Your guardian refuses to let you try the schooling. He says you never did much in school before, so it is a waste of time. He feels you are needed at home, and that is where you should be.

Difficulty getting married. You are 26 and want to get married. Your future spouse lives alone in an apartment. Your guardian does not feel you are ready to get married. Your guardian does not like your future spouse. You want to run off and get married. Some people tell you that you can, and others tell you your guardian can have the marriage annulled. Note: under current law, the marriage of the ward shall terminate the guardianship of the person, but not of the estate.

Difficulty getting a license. You move to the country and need to drive to a bus stop to get to work. You pass the tests but are refused a driver's license because you have a guardian. Your friend in the city has a license since the examiner did not know he has a guardian.

RIGHTS REMAINING WITH THE WARD

Guardians do have limits set by statute and court rulings. For example, the guardian may not force the ward to have an abortion, or undergo sterilization or electroshock therapy. The guardian cannot put the ward in an institution without court approval. The guardian cannot make a will for the ward, and cannot vote for the ward.

Since guardianship takes so many rights away from a person, courts always consider alternatives before imposing a guardianship. Everyone involved in a guardianship case should consider alternatives that maximize the person's independence and still ensure safety.

GUARDIANSHIP PROCESS

The following information is derived from materials prepared by the Ohio Association of Probate Judges. The information is very typical of situations in many states. Consult a lawyer for assistance with guardianship and alternatives.

What is a guardianship? A guardianship is an involuntary trust relationship in which one party, called the guardian, acts for an individual called a ward. The law regards the ward as incapable of managing their person and/or affairs.

What is a guardian? A guardian is any adult person, association, or corporation appointed by the probate court to assume responsibility for the care and management of the person, the estate, or both, of an incompetent person or minor child. A corporation can only be guardian of the estate and not of the person.

Types of guardians. A guardian may be appointed either a guardian of the person, a guardian of the estate, or both. A guardian of the person has custody of, controls, and protects the person of the ward. A guardian of the estate controls and protects the assets or property of the ward. A limited guardian may be appointed with limited powers to make restricted or specific decisions of the ward. The ward retains all powers not granted to the guardian.

Who needs a guardian? A guardian may be appointed for either an incompetent or minor, which are defined by statute. **Incompetent:** any person who is so mentally impaired as a result of a mental or physical illness or disability, or mental retardation, or as a result of chronic substance abuse, that he is incapable of taking proper care of himself or his property or fails to provide for his family or other persons for whom he is charged by law to provide, or any person confined to a penal institution within this state. **Minor:** any person under 18 years of age who has neither father nor mother or whose parents are unsuitable to have custody and tuition of such minor, or whose interests, in the opinion of the court, will be promoted. **Minor settlement:** natural parents do not have an inherent right to settle personal injury claims on behalf of a minor child. The probate court must authorize approval of such settlements. If the settlement exceeds $10,000, the Court will require the appointment of a guardian of an estate.

Who chooses the guardian? The court appoints the guardian. However, a minor over 14, or the parents by will, may suggest a guardian for a minor. In addition, an adult, while competent, may nominate a guardian to serve in the event of incapacity.

What is the appointment procedure? Application for guardianship is filed in the probate court of the county of the ward's residence by an interested party, or on the court's own motion. The application must include a statement of the guardian's willingness to perform as guardian, a bond as required by law, and, in the case of a prospective incompetent ward, a statement of the ward's mental and physical condition from a treating physician, psychiatrist, or licensed psychologist. The prospective ward, as well as the adult next of kin, will be notified of impending guardianship and date and time of hearing. In the case of an incompetent proceeding, the notice and a statement of rights will be served on the prospective ward by a court investigator. An investigation is conducted, in the case of a prospective incompetent ward, by a court investigator, which includes an interview with the prospective ward in order to assist the court in determining the advisability of guardianship. Formal hearing is conducted by the judge or referee to determine if a guardianship is necessary, the guardian is suitable, and the guardian understands his duties. **In an emergency** in which significant injury to a prospective ward may occur unless immediate action is taken, the court may appoint an emergency guardian for 72 hours.

What are the rights of the ward? The prospective ward has the right to be present at the hearing, to contest any application for guardianship, to have a record of the hearing taken, to have a friend or family member present at the hearing, and to be represented by an attorney. A prospective incompetent ward has the additional right to present evidence of a less restrictive alternative, and, if indigent and requested, to have an attorney and independent expert appointed at court expense.

Does the probate court have a supervisory role in the guardianship? The probate court is the superior guardian, and all guardians must obey all orders of the court. The court exerts its supervisory authority through accountings, periodic reports, and investigations. The court may order an investigation by a court investigator, law enforcement agency, adult protective service, or other county agency. The guardian must first obtain approval of the probate court before entering into contracts or leases, making improvement to real estate, mortgaging real estate, selling assets of the ward, or settling any personal injury claim for the ward. The court may, at any time, in the best interest of the ward, remove the guardian. A guardian's compensation and attorney's fees are set by court rule, and must be approved prior to fees being paid.

Terminating a guardianship. A court order will terminate a guardianship upon the death of a ward, upon the ward being adjudged competent, or, in the case of a minor, upon reaching the age of majority (18). In Ohio, a motion for termination of a guardianship of an incompetent may be filed 120 days after an appointment of a guardian, and once every year thereafter.

ALTERNATIVES TO GUARDIANSHIP

Every state has a menu of alternative methods used to support people who have difficulty managing their own affairs. Some require court action. Others are contracts or written documents that must be written up with certain formalities. A person must have legal capacity to enter into these arrangements. Obtain legal advice before proceeding with any of these arrangements.

CONSERVATORSHIP

A conservatorship is a voluntary trust relationship using guardianship laws and procedures as its basis, in which one party, known as a conservator, acts with court supervision for a competent, physically infirm adult, who is called the conservatee. A conservatorship is based on the consent of the person for whom the conservatorship is to benefit. Thus, the conservatee decides who will serve as conservator, and what property and powers of the conservatee will be included in the conservatorship. In addition, the conservatee decides which of the guardianship duties and procedures the conservator follows and the court enforces.

POWERS OF ATTORNEY

A power of attorney is written authorization for an agent to perform specified acts, either personal (healthcare) or estate (property) on behalf of a principal. There are several types of powers of attorney. **Durable powers of attorney** have powers that remain in effect in the event of the grantor's incapacity or on being adjudged incompetent. **Springing powers of attorney** become effective when the grantor becomes incapacitated or is adjudged incompetent. **Durable powers of attorney for health care** may be used to authorize healthcare decisions in the event of incapacity.

INTERVIVOS TRUSTS

An intervivos trust is a confidential relationship involving a trustee, who manages only the property of a living person for the benefit of that person or someone else. Substantial assets are usually needed to justify an intervivos trust arrangement.

ADVANCE DIRECTIVES

Advance directives are legal documents people can complete to express their wishes regarding their future healthcare. The forms and requirements are governed by state law. Even though standard forms are available, the choices on the forms are literally matters of life and death. Decisions should be well considered. Make sure you have sound advice.

People can use advance directives to guide their own care in the event that their attending physician determines that they lack capacity to make their own healthcare choices. Developing an advance directive offers people the opportunity to openly discuss signs and symptoms of illness, as well as treatment preferences. When properly planned and implemented, an advance directive is a natural expression of empowerment and recovery.

A declaration for mental health treatment may address issues like medications the person may or may not want to take, where treatment should be provided, preferences about types of treatment, and choices about temporary care of children or pets.

CRIMINAL JUSTICE SYSTEM

It is a sad fact that local jails have become the nation's largest source of inpatient psychiatric care. People incarcerated in local jails have rates of mental illnesses or substance abuse problems that are seven times greater than the rate of these illnesses in the general population. These rates are even higher in the juvenile justice system. A significant amount of mental illness in jails goes undetected even when correctional staff follows screening protocols at booking. Jail suicide is another serious problem, with rates well in excess of that in the general population.

Many law enforcement officers have not been appropriately trained to handle incidents involving people with mental illness. The standard police response involves coercive, stressful, command tactics that people with mental illness have difficulty processing. Responding to people with mental illness takes additional skills that may appear counterintuitive to police officers. These tactics seek to calm the individual, stabilize the situation, and reduce stress so the person can voluntarily comply with police requests. There is a developing consensus that police agencies should deploy these strategies, and that it may even be negligent not to do so. These crisis intervention strategies increase safety for everyone involved.

Many times, the family has called on law enforcement in response to a potentially volatile or self-destructive situation at home. Police have traditionally had just two options when they arrive on scene. They can arrest the person or transport the person to a mental health center for an evaluation. This evaluation could result in an involuntary emergency commitment to a state hospital or voluntary participation in inpatient or outpatient treatment. For a variety of reasons, police usually choose to arrest the person, resulting in the mentally ill person being detained in the local jail.

People with mental illness get stuck in jails. Conditions in jails for people with mental illness are generally horrific. Author Pete Earley has been investigating local jails for years. He wrote the following in August 2011.

> Put simply, the Miami Dade Pre-trial Detention Center is a living hell on earth for inmates with mental illnesses... If conditions at the Miami Dade jail were an aberration, then the rest of the country could simply shake its head, sigh, and sleep easy at night. But my travels to more than 46 states in the past five years have convinced me that the overcrowded and dangerous conditions that I observed in the Miami Dade County jail are not uncommon.

In September 2011, as part of an episode of the A&E Network television show *Beyond Scared Straight*, at-risk teens toured a suicide isolation cell in a Virginia jail, a room with padded walls and a clear plastic door. Correctional officers told the children that suicidal people were locked naked in the room with just a blanket. The toilet was the hole in the floor.

Unless the symptoms of mental illness are so severe that the person cannot be managed in the jail environment, evaluation and treatment will take place in jail at the convenience of correctional staff, with limited access to mental health staff. The best jails implement programs that connect inmates with case management agencies, and release prisoners for treatment in the community while they are awaiting trial.

ASSISTING A PERSON WHO HAS BEEN ARRESTED

When someone is booked into a jail, family members and friends can help make sure that the jail provides mental health treatment. It is particularly important to report any indications that the person may be suicidal. If you can, bring the person's medication to the jail.

Staff in the jail should perform an initial screening on everyone who is admitted to determine whether they are showing any symptoms of mental illness and if they have been receiving mental health treatment in the community. They should also screen for any risk factors for suicide. These screenings are usually brief. Sometimes people do not wish to disclose this information. Friends and family members who contact jail medical staff or jail administrators can provide information to support a more complete assessment that helps get better care.

Notify the person's case manager and other treatment providers about the incarceration. Case managers can help ensure continuation of treatment in jail, and can help support requests for bail or early release. Some mental health centers maintain formal lines of communication with the local jail, and have information sharing protocols that support coordinated mental health treatment.

In addition, a call to the incarcerated person's attorney may help secure a mental health evaluation and appropriate treatment. The attorney may also request that the court order an evaluation of the individual's competence to stand trial and/or mental condition at the time of the offense.

DIVERSION PROGRAMS

The prevailing model of justice system diversion is the so-called Sequential Intercept Model. This model recognizes that once a person enters the formal justice system pipeline, the person is at much higher risk of collateral consequences. At the very least, the person acquires an arrest record that will be accessible to future employers. Convictions can permanently restrict employment and even housing options. If the person moves far enough into the system, the person becomes subject to probation supervision, incarceration, and parole supervision.

The sequential intercept model identifies diversion opportunities at each step of justice system processing. Interception has several objectives: preventing initial involvement in the criminal justice system, decreasing admissions to jail, engaging individuals in treatment as soon as possible, minimizing time spent moving through the criminal justice system, linking individuals to community treatment upon release from incarceration, and decreasing the rate of return to the criminal justice system. Diversion programs are being implemented in many communities. These diversion alternatives are often reserved for mentally ill people accused of nonviolent misdemeanor offenses who would otherwise end up in jail for weeks or months.

The sequential intercept model diverts the most cases when cases are intercepted early. Preventing a person from having even minimal contact with law enforcement is the ultimate intercept. Any person not arrested avoids the collateral consequences of a criminal record. The later in the process the person is intercepted, the greater the collateral consequences.

Effective diversion prevents arrests and improves safety for everyone concerned. In the Crisis Intervention Team model, specially trained officers, and sometimes mental health professionals, are assigned to work the streets. When officers encounter a person whose conduct manifests signs of a mental illness, they have the option of taking the person to a mental health agency rather than to jail. The success of this kind of program depends upon the officers being able to recognize the signs of mental illness and on the capacity of the agency that has agreed to accept, evaluate, and engage individuals in treatment.

Because so few unruly individuals actually require inpatient hospitalization, some communities have set up respite centers that allow people to calm down and control their behavior. Some respites are peer-run. Community respite interrupts unruly behavior without burdening the criminal justice system. The alternative, the misdemeanor legal process, is often ineffective, even from the point of view of law enforcement, especially when jail space is limited. In many cities, unruly people are arrested and transported to jail, where they are given a court date and immediately released on their own recognizance. The court date is ignored, and an arrest warrant is issued. When people eventually appear in court, the judge releases them again.

Post-arrest diversion programs screen inmates and release individuals to their existing mental health agency or refer them for treatment. Depending on the kinds of arrangements that have been made between the mental health and criminal justice systems, the prosecutor may agree to drop the charges if the person agrees to participate in treatment. Sometimes judges may agree to grant probation with intensive mental health treatment instead of jail time. In many communities, the person's legal case may be referred to a mental health court or special docket where the judge has access to mental health staff and treatment resources. Treatment becomes a condition of probation, with goals of improving treatment compliance, stabilizing the person's daily life, and eliminating or reducing the amount of time spent in jail.

The sequential intercept model delivers increasingly coercive solutions as people move further into the court system. For example, pleading guilty to a charge in order to qualify for a "treatment court" program can sometimes increase a person's risk of incarceration, especially if there is a chance of winning the case. If the person has an addiction or mental health problem, refusing to accept particular forms of treatment or medication (ordinarily a person's right) can result in probation violations and incarceration. The promise that a conviction may be set aside upon program completion may never pay off, because most people who enter treatment courts have so-called "chronically relapsing" disorders and symptoms will almost certainly return at some point. On the other hand, a treatment court might be the very opportunity a person needs to address their difficulties and build their capacity for recovery. The key benefit of participation in a treatment court may be the opportunity to make positive human connections with peer mentors, judges, and attorneys.

RE-ENTRY PROGRAMS

Another critical point for people in the criminal justice system is re-entry. It is important that former prisoners returning to the community be promptly linked with appropriate treatment. Many people released from jail or prison remain under court supervision for a period of time. Probation and parole officers generally support appropriate treatment for the people in their caseloads. They assist in arranging appropriate treatment for people with mental illness.

Current research indicates that criminal behavior risk, mental health risk, and substance abuse risk are separate matters. Reducing reoffending involves reducing the criminal behavior risk directly. Addressing mental health or substance abuse does not have as much impact. Treatment for so-called criminogenic factors involves a specialized form of cognitive behavioral therapy.

PART FIVE
FOLLOWING YOUR PLAN

PLANNING FOR SUCCESS

Planning might sound like a technical, objective process, but there is also an emotional component. Make sure you stay connected to people as you do your planning work. If you start feeling over-whelmed, take a break. Remember that every human being faces difficult challenges at some point in life.

Strategic planning starts with one sheet of paper and four words.

- Strengths
- Weaknesses
- Opportunities
- Threats

Start your plan the same way. Use the four words as starting points for lists. You can work on all four areas simultaneously, or work one area at a time. Write whatever comes to mind. You do not need to write long essays. Find someone to help you if you get stuck.

STRENGTHS

Everyone has talents and capacities, even people with labels like "disabled" or "caregiver" or "mentally ill." What are your talents? What is your expertise?

You have gifts and talents you can use to benefit yourself or share with others. Start with what have you accomplished in the last week, the past few months or earlier in your life. What have you accomplished with some help and what did you rely on to succeed? What helps you handle stress? When are you best able to think? Who are the allies you have today in your family, community, neighborhood, or church? What economic resources do you have? Think about artistic ability, training you have had, the parts of your jobs that were successful. Sometimes depression takes the joy out of things you once enjoyed. Ignore the depression, and write those things down anyway.

IDENTIFY YOUR STRENGTHS

VIA Institute researchers have identified some two dozen key personal strengths valued by every culture on earth. VIA offers a free online test people can use to discover their own top character strengths. Learn more and take the VIA Strengths Survey at http://www.viame.org.

WEAKNESSES

Every human being has weaknesses. What are your weaknesses? You may not be able to handle physical tasks or emotional stress as well as you once did. You may need more sleep, or become fatigued more easily. Some situations may be difficult for you. You may have issues with transportation, isolation, money, housing, or relationships. Do not freak out by the size of your list. Everyone has a list. Addressing your weaknesses helps you start building up your own capacity.

OPPORTUNITIES

These are ways to turn your strengths, gifts, and capacities into action. What can you accomplish now, or accomplish with some help? Start with opportunities to connect with potential allies. As your allies open doors for you, your list of opportunities will grow. List potential allies even if you do not know how to connect with them or exactly what might happen later. For example, in your neighborhood or community there are libraries, parks, church groups and organizations you can connect with. Write these down. Do some online research. The NAMI and Mental Health America websites have information about support groups across the U.S. Track down the support groups in your area. Do not limit yourself to the clinical treatment system. What is in the larger community? Every publicly funded program works with people with mental health conditions. Recreation centers offer exercise classes and fitness activities that can keep you healthier or help relieve loneliness or depression. Advocacy groups can help you find housing, medical care or a job. You can participate in church activities and help others use their talents too. If you are a caregiver, you can connect with other caregivers. Type "caregiver assistance" in an internet search box, or get in touch with the home visit coordinator for your church or for a community elderly service program.

THREATS

You must identify the risks you face. What specific deadlines are you facing? What are you avoiding? This is hard, but identifying a threat is the first step to handling it. Consider John Carmody's universal toolkit for trouble: thinking, feeling, sharing, determination, and prayer. If you cannot handle this part alone, find an ally.

CREATE YOUR VISION

Your four lists help lay out your situation, your potential allies, resources you can access to move forward, plus the risks that you must deal with.

Let the lists sit for a day or so.

Continue your planning by answering ten questions about your vision for the future.

- What do you like to do?
- What do you do well?
- Who are the people who are important to you?
- What matters most to you?
- What are some places you like to go?
- What challenges do you face?
- What are your hopes, dreams, and desires?
- What do you want to do during the day?
- What do you want to do most this year?
- What things do you want to change this year?

EXTEND YOUR RANGE

Use the Safe Zone System to extend your range, and do more in your neighborhood or community. The Safe Zone System is a three-step process. The goal is to extend your range, access the whole world, and still stay safe.

1. Classify places and situations into zones.

- Zone One is home base or "recovery space," where there is maximum safety.

- Zone Two is "routine space," familiar places like work or school.

- Zone Three is "adventure space," places with higher stress or stimulation.

2. Do a capacity self-assessment. How am I doing right now?

3. Match capacity to space. Where can I be safe right now?

If you cannot be safe at the present zone level, move to the next lower zone or to recovery space. If you are having trouble in recovery space, contact someone for help.

TAKE ACTION

Action steps are next. What are one to three things you could do right away?

That is your plan.

Talk your answers over with somebody you trust.

Now get started.

BEYOND RECOVERY

Throughout this book, we have focused on recovery. Recovery was a revolutionary concept when it first emerged. It meant that people could make progress, get better, and control their own lives. This was a real affront to traditional thinking. Patients in locked asylums seldom had any choices.

But that was decades ago.

Recovery is now a mature concept. Treatment systems are adapting so they can better support recovery. That is not the end of it. We are learning it is possible for a person to move beyond recovery.

When people do what they must to stay healthy, pursue a focused process of recovery, see their doctor, keep connected to treatment and support, and manage their vulnerabilities and risks, they can do much more. People can flourish.

Flourishing means you can use all your strengths and capacities, do well, live a full life, have a family, participate in your community, and succeed in your work. You can be effective.

You can find your element, the place where the things you are good at and the things you love to do come together. You can use your strengths to do the things you love.

What are you good at? What do you love to do?

Our culture sometimes makes it hard to recognize our strengths. Sir Ken Robinson's book *The Element* talks about how our educational system values one or two kinds of human potential over all the others. First graders get grades for math, but not for dancing or being social or kind. After years of this, we develop blind spots about our talents and about what matters to us. We can find our strengths, and recognize what brings us joy, but we must be willing to look.

Everyone has strengths and limitations. Creating a successful future involves paying attention to both. As you move beyond recovery and into your element, you must pay due attention to your limits. You may have wobbly moods and a collection of medical issues. You certainly have your own faults and hang-ups. You may need to take your medicine. You will not be able to accomplish everything you attempt.

However, you can choose to work on goals that are not connected to your illness. You can have an identity and a future not determined by your diagnosis or whatever might be published in a future volume of the DSM.

Recovery gets you through the struggle of mental illness. However, there is more to life than that.

You can take all the skills you ever had, plus new skills you have learned in recovery, and complete your larger journey.

You can find your element, and flourish.

MENTAL HEALTH RECOVERY EVERYWHERE

Mental illness is a problem throughout the population. Mental health issues lurk behind every failure rate in our society, and behind our most shocking tragedies. Every month, over 3,000 Americans die by suicide. One in five Americans has experienced severe mental distress in the past 30 days.

The US mental health treatment system needs backup. We know it does not reach everyone. It is designed to be expensive, with professional care that can reach just one person at a time, even when the system is working at its best. We actually disable the rest of society when we say that only clinical solutions can help. That is blind-spot thinking, half a step past shunning and exclusion.

Let's make a different sort of commitment to addressing mental health. Let's activate everyone. We can put mental health recovery everywhere, with nonclinical support that stands next to the clinical system. The two can work together.

All we need to get started are a few examples of people stepping forward, putting aside their customary denials and defensive thinking, and finding opportunities to help each other. There is a place in our society for nonclinical support and outreach work.

Friends and family members are actually doing this now, in every neighborhood across America. We just need these efforts to go public. Churches, businesses, community groups, neighborhood clinics, veteran's organizations, schools, colleges, and fitness centers can get many more people started. What if every group that uses volunteers spent an hour a year on mental health support training?

Everyone can learn to ask a few questions and help a friend.

Until Alcoholics Anonymous was invented in the early 1930s, the world had no solutions for addiction. Today there are 66,000 nonclinical addiction recovery groups meeting in church basements, libraries, and community centers across America. Volunteers help people start their recovery, and help people stay sober, no matter how much damage a person has sustained over the course of his addiction. AA made addiction approachable.

With *Defying Mental Illness,* there's a way to do the same for mental health. This book is fully compatible with clinical systems. Your group can shatter the myths that disempower people, and turn worried bystanders into allies. You can help people talk through what they are facing, and support your friends, and help keep everyone safe.

Finally, there is a way to pitch in.

Let's get started.

ACKNOWLEDGMENTS

My wife Esther and my children Andrew, Peter, and Sophia showed me the power of love and support despite everything.

Andrea Schroer pushed so much hope into this work, and encouraged me to make it personal.

Peter Block taught me to focus on how communities work, and how to envision possibilities and gifts. I appreciate the opportunity to work and to learn from him, as well as his support of this project. Peter even taught me how to autograph my books.

I appreciate the advice, wisdom, encouragement and support I have received from so many people. Special thanks to Milt Greek, Rex Lai, Corinna West, Malaika Puffer, Patty Roeding, Tina Michel, Maggie Campbell-Reynolds, Gayle Hilleke, Sharon Sapienz, Diane Rogers, Dr. Jeremy Engel, Bonnie Hedrick, Ann Barnum, Dr. Fred Frese, Sunnie Southern, Barry Isaacs, Marilyn Hyland, and Sarah Hyland. I wish more of my readers could have met my departed friends Dr. Sung Kim and Jenny Edwards. Dr. Kim taught me Chinese medicine, complexity, and systems thinking. Jenny was the personification of badass joy, courage, and commitment.

I have also learned from my readers and the people I have corresponded with on LinkedIn, Facebook, and Twitter, especially Randye Kaye, Barbara Altman, Debbie Corso, Guy Gambill, Lorna d'Entremont, Andy Behrman, and Dr. Michelle Golland.

I know I am leaving out 20,000 other names. So many people have helped me or taught me, or shared their struggles with me. I apologize for the omissions. I am so much better at being grateful than I am at remembering names.

Thank you all so much.

— Paul Komarek

APPENDIX STRATEGIES AND TOOLS

THE STRATEGY FOR RECOVERY

1. Learn about what you are facing.

2. Find allies to support you.

3. Find resources to work with.

4. Plan both near-term and long-term.

5. Follow your plan.

FOUR QUESTIONS FOR RECOVERY

1. What helps you make the most of your talents?

2. How can you reduce the areas where you are vulnerable?

3. How can you improve your ability to cope with stress?

4. How can you deal with the risk of something going wrong?

FOUR QUESTIONS AMONG FRIENDS

1. What have you accomplished since the last time we met?

2. What are you facing?

3. Who are your allies?

4. What is your plan?

THE SAFE ZONE SYSTEM

The Safe Zone System is a three-step process.

1. Classify places and situations into zones.

- Zone One is home base or "recovery space," where there is maximum safety.

- Zone Two is "routine space," familiar places like work or school.

- Zone Three is "adventure space," places with higher stress or stimulation.

2. Do a capacity self-assessment. How am I doing right now?

3. Match capacity to space. Where can I be safe right now?

If you cannot be safe at the present zone level, move to the next lower zone or to recovery space. If you are having trouble in recovery space, contact someone for help.

BIBLIOGRAPHY

Allen, K. E. (2007). *Developmental Profiles: Pre-Birth Through Twelve* (5th ed.). Clifton Park, NY: Thomson/Delmar Learning.

American Association of Suicidology. (2008). Suicide and Eating Disorders. Downloaded 9/4/2011 from http://www.suicidology.org.

Arc of New Jersey. (2010). Suspects with developmental disabilities and the criminal justice system.

Bakalar, N. (2013.). Delusions, Anger and Violence - NYTimes.com. Retrieved December 5, 2013, from http://well.blogs.nytimes.com/2013/03/11/delusions-anger-and-violence/?smid=tw-nytimeswell&seid=auto&pagewanted=print&_r=0

Balmert, J. (2013). Housing options for people with mental health issues vary greatly across Ohio. Zanesville Times Recorder. Retrieved December 5, 2013, from http://www.zanesvilletimesrecorder.com/article/BA/20130615/NEWS01/306150001/Housing-options-people-mental-health-issues-vary-greatly-across-Ohio

Barber, C. (2009). *Comfortably Numb: How Psychiatry Is Medicating a Nation*. New York: Vintage Books.

Becker, G. de. (1999). *The Gift of Fear and Other Survival Signals that Protect Us From Violence*. Dell.

Behrman, A. (2003). *Electroboy: a memoir of mania*. New York: Random House Trade Paperbacks.

Block, P. (2002). *The Answer to How Is Yes: Acting on What Matters*. San Francisco, CA: Berrett-Koehler Publishers.

Block, P. (2008). *Community the structure of belonging*. San Francisco: Berrett-Koehler Publishers.

Borderline Personality Disorder. (2011). Retrieved September 19, 2011, from http://www.borderlinepersonalitydisorder.com.

Brené Brown: Listening to shame | Video on TED.com. (2012). Retrieved from http://www.ted.com/talks/brene_brown_listening_to_ shame.html

Brené Brown: The power of vulnerability | Video on TED.com. (2010). Retrieved from http://www.ted.com/talks/brene_brown_on_vulnerabi lity.html

Brown, C. B. (2007). *I thought it was just me: women reclaiming power and courage in a culture of shame*. New York: Gotham.

Brown, C. B. (2010). *The gifts of imperfection: let go of who you think you're supposed to be and embrace who you are*. Center City, Minn: Hazelden.

Campbell, A. (1993). *Men, Women, and Aggression*. New York, NY: Basic Books.

Carmody, J. (1993). *How to Handle Trouble*. New York: Doubleday.

Carter, R. (1994). *Helping Yourself Help Others: A Book for Caregivers*. New York: Times Books.

Carter, R. (1998). *Helping Someone with Mental Illness: A Compassionate Guide for Family, Friends, and Caregivers*. New York: Times Books.

Carter, R., Golant, S. K., & Cade, K. E. (2010). *Within Our Reach: Ending the Mental Health Crisis* (1st ed.). Rodale Books.

Chamberlin, J. (1978). *On our own: Patient-controlled alternatives to the mental health system* (Second Print.). Hawthorn Books.

Coleman, R. (2011). *Recovery: An Alien Concept?* (3rd Revised ed.). P & P Press.

Corbett, S. (2009). *When Helping Hurts: How to Alleviate Poverty Without Hurting the Poor — and Yourself*. Chicago, IL: Moody Publishers.

Corso, D., Smith, A., & Paz, A. (2012). *Stop Sabotaging: A 31 Day DBT Challenge to Change Your Life*.

Council of State Governments Justice Center. (2002). *Criminal Justice / Mental Health Consensus Project*. New York: Author.

Council of State Governments Justice Center. (2011). http://www.justicecenter.csg.org/

Courtade, R. (2008). *Self-help for Fear and Anger: The Recovery Method*. Createspace.

Cozolino, L. (2013). *The social neuroscience of education: optimizing attachment and learning in the classroom*. New York: Norton.

Daalmans, J. (2013). The Complexity of Cultural Change, Pt. 1. SciTech Connect. Retrieved December

5, 2013, from
http://scitechconnect.elsevier.com/complexity-
cultural-change-pt-1/

Daalmans, J. (2013). The Complexity of Cultural
Change, Pt. 2. SciTech Connect. Retrieved December
5, 2013, from
http://scitechconnect.elsevier.com/complexity-
cultural-change-pt-2/

Earley, P. (2006). *Crazy : A Father's Search Through
America's Mental Health Madness*. New York: G.P.
Putnam's Sons.

e-Patient Dave. http://epatientdave.com/

Fauteux, K. (2011). *Defusing angry people: practical
tools for handling bullying, threats, and violence.* Far
Hills, N.J.: New Horizon Press.

Figueroa, A. (2013). Dying for Company: Social Isolation Increases Death Risk in Older People. AlterNet.
Retrieved from http://www.alternet.org/personal-
health/dying-company-social-isolation-increases-
death-risk-older-
peo-
ple?akid=10245.1076401.TCFtJS&rd=1&src=newslet
ter815829&t=19

Freire, P. (2001). *Pedagogy of the oppressed.* New
York: Continuum.

Freire, P., & Freire, P. (1974). *Education for critical
consciousness.* London: Continuum.

Gershon, D. (2009). *Social change 2.0: a blueprint for
reinventing our world.* West Hurley, NY: High Point.

Goldsmith, S. (2002). *Reducing Suicide: A National Imperative*. Washington, DC: National Academies Press.

Goodwin, F. and Jamison, K. (1990). *Manic-Depressive Illness*. New York: Oxford University Press.

Grace, E. (2013). Cognitively Accessible Language (Why We Should Care). The Feminist Wire. Retrieved December 5, 2013, from http://thefeministwire.com/2013/11/cognitively-accessible-language-why-we-should-care/

Greek, M. (2010). How a Series of Hallucinations Tells a Symbolic Story. *Schizophrenia Bulletin* vol. 36 no. 6, pp. 1063-1065.

Greek, M. (2010). *Schizophrenia: A Blueprint for Recovery* http://www.schizophreniablueprint.com

Greek, M. (2012). *Schizophrenia: A Blueprint for Recovery*. CreateSpace Independent Publishing Platform.

Grohol, J. (2012). Top 25 Psychiatric Medication Prescriptions for 2011 - Psych Central. Psych Central.com. Retrieved December 5, 2013, from http://psychcentral.com/lib/top-25-psychiatric-medication-prescriptions-for-2011/00012586

Grossman, D. (2009). *On Killing: The Psychological Cost of Learning to Kill in War and Society*. New York: Little, Brown and Co.

Hallowell, E. & Ratey, J. (1994). *Driven to Distraction: Recognizing and Coping with Attention Deficit Disorder from Childhood Through Adulthood*. New York: Touchstone.

Harper, J. (2013). Bullying, Mobbing and the Role of Shame. Retrieved December 5, 2013, from http://www.psychologytoday.com/blog/beyond-bullying/201309/bullying-mobbing-and-the-role-shame

Hobson, J. A. (1994). *The Chemistry of Conscious States: How the Brain Changes Its Mind.* Boston: Little, Brown.

Jamison, K. R. (1995). *An Unquiet Mind.* New York: Knopf.

Jamison, K. R. (1999). *Night Falls Fast: Understanding Suicide.* New York: Knopf.

Jantz, Gregory. (2010). *Hope, Help & Healing for Eating Disorders.* Colorado Springs, CO: WaterBrook Press

Joiner, T. E. (2007). *Why people die by suicide.* Cambridge, Mass.: Harvard University Press.

Judd, Sandra. ed. (2011). *Eating Disorders Sourcebook.* 3rd Edition. Detroit, MI: Omnigraphics.

Kaiser Commission on Medicaid and the Uninsured.(2005). Medicaid: An Overview of Spending on "Mandatory" vs. "Optional" Populations and Services Washington, DC: Henry J. Kaiser Family Foundation.

Kaye, R. (2011). B*en Behind His Voices: One Family's Journey from the Chaos of Schizophrenia to Hope.* Rowman & Littlefield Publishers.

Ken Robinson: Changing education paradigms | Video on TED.com. (n.d.). Retrieved from http://www.ted.com/talks/ken_robinson_changing_ed ucation_paradigms.html

Komarek, P. (2001). *Working with People with Mental Illness in the Criminal Justice System*. Columbus, OH: NAMI Ohio.

Komarek, P. (2004). *You Are Not Alone: Mental Illness, Community Resources, Family Supports*. Columbus, OH: NAMI Ohio.

Komarek, P. (2012). Redesigning Mental Illness. http://redesigningmentalillness.blogspot.com.

Komarek, P. (2012, December 13). Mass murder is the new flavor of American suicide. Redesigning Mental Illness. Retrieved from http://redesigningmentalillness.blogspot.com/2012/12 /mass-murder-is-new-flavor-of-american.html

Komarek, P. (2013, November 26). Adam Lanza's suicide ignored by state report. Retrieved December 5, 2013, from http://redesigningmentalillness.blogspot.com/2013/11 /adam-lanzas-suicide-ignored-by-state.html

Kretzmann, J. and McKnight, J. (1993). *Building Communities from the Inside Out: A Path Toward Finding and Mobilizing a Community's Assets*. Chicago, IL: ACTA Publications.

Lankford, A. (2013). *The myth of martyrdom: what really drives suicide bombers, rampage shooters, and other self-destructive killers*. New York, NY: Palgrave Macmillan.

Low, A. A., & Low, A. A. (1997). *Mental Health Through Will Training: A System of Self-Help in Psy-*

chotherapy As Practiced by Recovery, Incorporated (3rd ed.). Willett Pub Co.

Lustbader, W. (1991). *Counting on Kindness: The Dilemmas of Dependency.* New York: Free Press.

Lustbader, W. (2001). *What's Worth Knowing.* New York: Tarcher/Putnam.

McKnight, J. and Block, P. (2010). *The Abundant Community: Awakening the Power of Families and Neighborhoods.* San Francisco: Berrett-Koehler Publishers.

Medicare Premiums, deductibles and copays. http://www.medicareadvocacy.org/2011/10/27/2012-medicare-premiums-deductibles-and-co-pays/

Medicare Rights Center (2006). Clearing Hurdles and Hitting Walls: Restrictions Undermine Part D Coverage of Mental Health Drugs. Downloaded 8/26/12 from http://www.medicarerights.org/issues-actions/publications.php.

Medicare Rights Center. (2006). Medicare Drug Plans Should Lift Restrictions on Mental Health Drugs. Downloaded 8/24/12 from http://www.medicarerights.org/issues-actions/publications.php#

Mental Health America. http://www.nmha.org/

Miller, B. (2013). Health law may strain mental health system. Retrieved December 5, 2013, from http://www.usatoday.com/story/news/nation/2013/11/03/health-law-may-strain-mental-health-system/3398593/

Minnesota Department of Human Services. (2012). Co-occurring Disorders Integrated Dual Disorders Treatment IDDT MN ver2. Retrieved December 5, 2013, from http://www.dhs.state.mn.us/main/idcplg?IdcService= GET_DYNAMIC_CONVERSION&dID=119908

NAMI: National Alliance on Mental Illness. http://www.nami.org/

National Institute on Drug Abuse (NIDA). (2013). Retrieved December 5, 2013, from http://www.drugabuse.gov/

National Prevention Council. (2011). *National Prevention Strategy.* Washington, DC: U.S. Department of Health and Human Services, Office of the Surgeon General.

National Research Council and Institute of Medicine. (2000). *From Neurons to Neighborhoods: The Science of Early Childhood Development.* Washington, DC: National Academy Press.

Network of Care. (2011). http://www.networkofcare.org

Neugeboren, J. (1999). *Transforming Madness: New Lives for People Living with Mental Illness.* New York: William Morrow & Company.

NYAPRS : Peer Bridger Project. (2010). Retrieved September 10, 2011, from http://www.nyaprs.org/peer-services/peer-bridger/

Paul, A. M. (2013). From The Brilliant Report: A Surprising Way To Improve Executive Function « Annie Murphy Paul. Retrieved December 5, 2013, from http://anniemurphypaul.com/2013/03/from-the-brilliant-report-a-surprising-way-to-improve-executive-function/

Payne, R. K. (2005). *A Framework for Understanding Poverty*. Highlands, TX: Aha! Process.

Payne, R. K. (2006). *Bridges Out of Poverty: Strategies for Professionals and Communities*. Highlands, TX: aha! Process.

Perry, Bruce. (1996) Neurodevelopmental Adaptations To Violence: How Children Survive The Intragenerational Vortex Of Violence. Downloaded 2/3/13 from http://www.childtrauma.org/ctamaterials/vortex_violence.asp

Pinker, S. (1997). *How the Mind Works*. New York, NY: Norton.

Pinker, S. (2002). *The Blank Slate: The Modern Denial of Human Nature*. New York, NY: Viking.

Pinker, S. (2010). *The Better Angels of Our Nature: Why Violence Has Declined* (F First Edition edition.). Viking Adult.

Pipher, M. B. (2013). *The green boat: reviving ourselves in our capsized culture.*

Porter, R. (2002). *Madness: A Brief History*. Oxford: New York: Oxford University Press.

Powers, Richard E. (2005) Assessment And Management Of Aggressive Behavior For The Person With Intellectual Disability. Downloaded 2/3/13 from www.ddmed.org/pdfs/2.pdf.

PTSD Overview — National Center for PTSD. (2011). Retrieved September 19, 2011, from http://www.ptsd.va.gov/public/pages/fslist-ptsd-overview.asp.

Queensland Alliance. (2010). *From discrimination to social inclusion: A review of the literature on anti-stigma initiatives in mental health.* Downloaded from www.qldalliance.org.au

Ratey, J. and Cameron, J. (1997). *Shadow Syndromes.* New York: Pantheon Books.

Rath, T. (2007). *Strengthsfinder 2.0.* Omaha: Gallup Press : [distributor] Grantham Book Services Ltd.

Resnick, P. (2010). *Risk Assessment for Violence.* Presentation materials August/September 2010, Cleveland, OH.

Robinson, K., & Aronica, L. (2009). *The Element: How Finding Your Passion Changes Everything* (Reprint.). Penguin Books.

Rosenberg, T. (2012). *Join the Club: How Peer Pressure Can Transform the World.* Icon Books.

Schiller, L. (1994). *The Quiet Room: A Journey Out of the Torment of Madness.* New York: Warner Books.

Schneier, B. (2003). *Beyond Fear: Thinking Sensibly About Security in an Uncertain World.* Springer.

Search Institute. (2011). *What Kids Need: The Building Blocks for Children and Youth.* Retrieved September 24, 2011, from http://www.search-institute.org/developmental-assets.

Semeniuk, I. (2013). How poverty influences a child's brain development. The Globe and Mail. Retrieved December 5, 2013, from http://www.theglobeandmail.com/technology/science/

brain/how-poverty-influences-a-childs-brain-development/article7882957/

Shera, D. W. (Ed.). (2003). *Emerging Perspectives on Anti-Oppressive Practice*. Canadian Scholars Press.

Shirky, C. (2008). *Here comes everybody: the power of organizing without organizations*. New York: Penguin Press.

Solomon, A. (2001). *The Noonday Demon: An Atlas of Depression*. New York: Scribner.

Spring, C. (2013). Coping with crisis - dealing with dissociation. Retrieved December 5, 2013, from http://www.pods-online.org.uk/copingwithcrisis.html

States Crack Down On Mental Health Prescriptions - Disability Scoop. (2012). Retrieved August 27, 2012, from http://www.disabilityscoop.com/2012/08/15/states-crack-down-prescriptions/16257/

Styron, W. (1992). *Darkness Visible: A Memoir of Madness*. New York: Vintage Books.

The Merck Manual of Medical Information. (2007). New York: Pocket Books.

Thirteen/WNET New York. (2001). *The Secret Life of the Brain*.

Thomas, S. (2013). Mental health and addiction parity: Four ways new rules will affect patients. The Grand Rapids Press - MLive.com. Retrieved December 5, 2013, from http://www.mlive.com/news/grand-rapids/index.ssf/2013/11/mental_health_and_addiction_pa.html

Toews, B. (2006). *The little book of restorative justice for people in prison: rebuilding the web of relationships.* Intercourse, PA: Good Books.

Tough, P. (2012). *How children succeed: grit, curiosity, and the hidden power of character.*

Tovar, V. (2013). Stigma Loading: The Effects of Disease Classification & AMA's Decision to Call Fat a Disease. Virgie Tovar: Hate Loss Not Weight Loss. Retrieved December 5, 2013, from http://www.virgietovar.com/2/post/2013/06/stigma-loading-the-effects-of-disease-classification-amas-decision-to-call-fat-a-disease.html

U.S. Department of Health and Human Services. (1999). *Mental Health: A Report of the Surgeon General* Rockville, MD: Author.

U.S. Department of Health and Human Services. (2002). *Report to Congress on the Prevention and Treatment of Co-Occurring Substance Abuse Disorders and Mental Disorders.* Rockville, MD: Author

U.S. Department of Health and Human Services. (2003). *Preventing Drug Use Among Children and Adolescents, A Research-Based Guide.* Rockville, MD: Author.

Whitaker, R. (2002). *Mad in America: Bad Science, Bad Medicine, and the Enduring Mistreatment of the Mentally Ill.* Cambridge, MA: Perseus Pub.

Whiteman, H. (2013). Depression affects memory by "impairing ability to differentiate similarities." Medical News Today. Retrieved December 5, 2013, from http://www.medicalnewstoday.com/articles/267039.php

Whybrow, P. C. (1997). *A Mood Apart: Depression, Mania, and Other Afflictions of the Self*. New York, NY: Basic Books.

Wolin, S. J., & Wolin, S. (1993). *The resilient self: how survivors of troubled families rise above adversity*. New York: Villard Books.

Wright, P. W. D. (2007). *Wrightslaw: Special Education Law* (2nd ed.). Hartfield, VA: Harbor House Law Press.

Wright, P. W. D. (2008). *Wrightslaw: From Emotions to Advocacy: The Special Education Survival Guide*. Hartfield, VA: Harbor House Law Press.

ABOUT THE AUTHORS

PAUL KOMAREK

Paul Komarek is an author, speaker, and consultant with a comeback story. After bipolar disorder wiped out his legal career, Paul rebuilt his life around his strengths as a writer, teacher, and policy expert. He works on tough social issues, including criminal justice reform, education of children with disabilities, violence prevention, addiction treatment, and healthcare for the poor.

Mr. Komarek is an adjunct faculty member at Cincinnati State Technical and Community College.

Learn more at **www.paulkomarek.us**.

Connect with Paul Komarek on Twitter **@pkomarek**.

Paul Komarek's blog project is **Redesigning Mental Illness www.redesigningmentalillness.net**

ANDREA SCHROER

Andrea Schroer is a teacher and educational consultant who assists schools, non-profit organizations, and businesses in reaching self-sufficiency through recommendations and training in the areas of tutor-

ing, after school programming, and child care licen-
sure.

Learn more at
http://www.supporttheireducation.com.

CHURCH BASEMENT PRESS

Church Basement Press publishes books that support the work of faith-based and community organizations and help people make progress in their lives.

To order additional copies of this and other Church Basement Press titles as an ebook, visit us on Smashwords.com.

www.smashwords.com/profile/view/churchbasement

For news about Church Basement Press titles, join our mailing list at **www.churchbasement.net**

Updates and Downloads

Our website includes helpful videos, downloadable worksheets, and links to additional resources. **www.DefyingMentalIllness.net**

Keep in touch with *Defying Mental Illness* on Facebook. **www.facebook.com/defyingmi**

Follow Paul Komarek on Twitter **@pkomarek**

CPSIA information can be obtained at www.ICGtesting.com
Printed in the USA
LVOW06s2154130314

377373LV00010B/165/P